Postnatal Depression

Vivienne Welburn was born near Scarborough in 1941, during the blackout. Because her parents worked abroad, she was educated from the age of nine at a Methodist girls' boarding school in Yorkshire. She later graduated from Leeds University and London University Institute of Education and worked for eight years as a teacher of English in London comprehensive schools.

She started writing when she was nine and wrote her first play at the age of eighteen. For the next twelve years she continued to write exclusively for the theatre. She has since branched out into journalism and book writing. Her first professional production was at the Traverse Theatre Club in Edinburgh in 1965. Her published plays are *Johnny So Long* and *The Drag* (1967); *Clearway* (1967); *The Treadwheel* and *Coil without Dreams* (1975). She also contributed to *Play Ten*, a book of short plays for schools (1977).

Vivienne Welburn currently works as a freelance writer. She lives in Chiswick with her husband (an administrator and poet) and her two daughters Imogen and Pippa.

VIVIENNE WELBURN

Postnatal Depression

FONTANA PAPERBACKS

First published by Fontana Paperbacks 1980
Copyright © Vivienne Welburn 1980

Set in Linotype Times

Made and printed in Great Britain by
William Collins Sons & Co. Ltd, Glasgow

For Imogen and Pippa, my daughters

Contents

Acknowledgements

My sincere gratitude must go first and foremost to all the women who talked to me, willingly and without recompense. Without them it would have been impossible to write this book. My thanks also to Christine Hankinson and Sally Partington for their hospitality on my travels out of London.

I would also like to thank the National Childbirth Trust (NCT), the Association for Improvements in Maternity Services (AIMS) and Depressives Associated for help and advice given, and also the doctors, psychiatrists, health visitors, antenatal teachers and social workers whose professional opinions and advice have been invaluable.

My deepest personal thanks for help and care during my depression go to Ann Hawker, Richard Stone, Pam Fawcett and Di and Mike Bartlett; also to Glynn Christian for endless babysitting during that period.

I am profoundly grateful to all the women who worked to ensure that my children were well cared for whilst I was busy working on this book, most especially their granny, Lea, who gave her time unstintingly; to Brigid Hanbury for her criticisms and typing of the manuscript; and to Giles Gordon for all his efforts on my behalf.

Above all my special thanks to Dulan Barber for rebuilding my professional confidence with endless reassurance, advice and criticism; and to my husband, Richard, for his faith, love and the many marvellous meals he cooked for me during the writing of this book.

Author's Note

I have given references for all material quoted from sources other than my own interviews.

Puerperal means of or due to childbirth. It derives from the Latin *puer* - boy, *pario* - to bear. Puerperal depression is the technical name for postnatal depression.

Contrary to custom I have chosen to describe babies and children as 'she' for the very personal reason that I have two daughters. I hope that parents of sons will take it as understood that I mean 'he' or 'she'.

Preface

In 1974, nine weeks after the birth of my second child, I became very depressed. I had never suffered from any kind of breakdown before and could not understand why this had happened. I turned to bookshops and libraries seeking information and found none, except for occasional paragraphs in some child-care and childbirth books assuring me that depression of this kind was rare. My doctor told me it was very common.

As I slowly moved up and out of my depression, two steps forward, one step back, I again took up my professional work as a writer. I started a number of projects, one of which was my own analysis of postnatal depression which has led to the writing of this book. As I moved into the community and talked to women I became impressed and disturbed by the extent of the problem. I realized that compared to many others' my own experience had been mild and my treatment excellent.

I felt it was important to present the wide range of experiences which constitute postnatal depression and talk to women in other areas of the country as well as London. I recorded and transcribed interviews with twenty-five women of different ages and social backgrounds in and around London, Leeds and Oxford, and must have talked informally to three times that number. In addition I received a number of letters from readers of *Mother and Baby* magazine as a result of a request for information published there. These women are not a representative sample in any scientific sense for this is not a scientific book; they are women who have talked willingly to me about a very painful and difficult period in their lives in the hope that their experiences may help other women. To protect their privacy I have, of course, altered all identifying names and places.

My intention is to stimulate discussion about and create awareness of this hidden problem and to assure those struggling through it that they are not alone: there are thousands of women who understand exactly how they feel.

As far as the professionals are concerned, I have consulted many and their opinions have been diverse.

1. *Misconceptions*

I am haunted by the image of Sylvia Plath in the months before her death, rising at four a.m. to write her poetry before her children woke and she embarked on a day's hard work mothering. What sort of society do we live in that requires a woman to drive herself to breaking point if she is to care adequately for her children *and* fulfil her own needs! We can only react as the people we are, not the eternal martyrs we are expected to be.

The misconceptions which surround the mother role are probably more damaging than those surrounding any of the other roles society expects women to play. Before she becomes a mother it is possible for a woman to be an intelligent companion, an efficient housewife, a well-groomed career woman, a superb cook and a multi-orgasmic lover. Once her baby is born she is in conflict with all the other roles, especially the sexual one. The mother-lover clash creates so much misery because it is unexpected and very deep rooted.

Sensuous and maternal have been created into opposing feminine images. The sensuous woman is fascinating to men and receives considerable publicity. What concerns me in this book, and what should concern men far more, are the ways in which the conventional virtues of motherhood can destroy the vitality and potential of the sensuous woman. As one young husband put it: 'I married a lovely sexy girl – then she turned into someone's mother.'[1]

The problem with the reproductive process has always been that you cannot have babies without having sex. Sex, however, is pleasurable and therein lies the dilemma. Having contorted themselves over the problem for hundreds of years, moralists, philosophers and medical men finally separated the sexual and reproductive functions of woman very successfully and created a dual sexual morality which required the opposing female roles of the whore and the mother, the good woman and the bad woman, sacred and profane love.

Dylan Thomas humorously portrays the dilemma in his play, *Under Milk Wood*, in the characters of Mrs Dai Bread One and Mrs Dai Bread Two, the wanton gypsy and the mumsy housewife. This is one solution to the problem and could well be part of the reason why men take mistresses. It is no solution for women though.

The image of the whore is sexual, exciting and despised. She is pursued by men as a sex object, a status symbol. It is not an uncommon plight for such women to find great difficulty in being maternal; Brigitte Bardot may be an example of this: international sex symbol, she abandoned her son in his infancy to be reared by his father. Perhaps she identified herself too closely with the stereotype she plays. On the other hand the image of the mother is virtually sexless: she is a responsible, respectable homemaker, not an ecstatic lover. It is a powerful image because we identify it with our own mothers whom we cannot imagine as sexual. But it also springs from the practical domestic situation.

The exclusive emphasis in our society on the *mother*-baby bond as the basis for mental health creates in us a constant 'on-call' consciousness. We must be alert for danger or distress signals day and night. This is not conducive to a successful sex life. Which of us has not made love with half an ear open for the baby's cry or the worry that our four-year-old might walk in? Which of us has not felt decidedly more sexually abandoned on that precious weekend away without the children?

There is also the combined effect of boredom and physical exhaustion. Most of the jobs connected with housework and infant care are physically arduous: washing, ironing, shopping, cleaning; lifting up, putting down and carrying something most of the day. But none of them requires much concentration or inspires interest. The excitement and involvement with life needed to stimulate sexual appetite just doesn't exist. While some headway has been made towards accepting the sensuous woman as normal and healthy (though preferably within marriage), almost no headway has been made towards releasing the maternal woman from continued and unremitting self-sacrifice.

The existence of the whore/mother stereotypes is based on a repressive morality and ensures that women are reared to be domestic *not* sexual. Premarital sex is still regarded with deep suspicion and anxiety by most parents. Most mothers actively discourage their daughters' sexual awareness, as their mothers did to them and their grandmothers did to their mothers and so on. This lack of sex education in the home inevitably leads girls to feel there must be something rather nasty about the whole thing. Whilst greater permissiveness in sexual behaviour is tolerated privately, public attitudes are still Victorian.

It is popular to talk about the repressions of Victorian morality as if they existed a thousand years ago. They didn't; the Victorians were our grandparents or great grandparents. The 1950s are already being treated as history while women from the suffragette movement are still alive to tell their tale and time concertinas with their memories. When I was thirteen my aunt warned me that I would drop dead, like one poor girl she knew, if I stood in bare feet on a cold floor when I had my period. If menstruation taboos die hard, so too does the dual morality.

A meeting of the Townswomen's Guilds in 1975 expressed deep concern about the moral dangers to which young girls were exposed – there was, needless to say, no corresponding concern about young boys. The general belief behind the dual morality is that sex is bestial and socially dangerous; that men are incapable of self-control sexually and women, being purer, are capable of infinite self-control. Therefore, all the ills which beset our permissive society can be blamed on women. The sanctions traditionally operated to support this code are the spread of VD, pregnancy as punishment and withholding marriage prospects from women who transgress.

Pregnancy as punishment is the ultimate deterrent in the moral conditioning of young girls for it is proof of immoral and loose behaviour. The conditioning is so strong that it reaches over into marriage and approved pregnancy. The most common verb for conception is 'fell' – fell pregnant, fell for a baby as in fell from grace, fallen woman:

the anti-sex connotations are sadly obvious. In Dickens's *David Copperfield* the only way Little Emily could survive the shame of being seduced by Steerforth (even though she was not pregnant) was to emigrate with her uncle to Australia. Today the unmarried girl who 'gets herself pregnant' (what happened to the man?) is socially ostracized, disgraces her parents and shocks the neighbours. If she lives in the provinces she may well flee to the anonymity of London. The emphasis is on the shame of being caught, not on the tragedy of an unwanted conception.

Boys, on the other hand, are tacitly encouraged to sow their wild oats. A man who is a virgin when he marries had better keep quiet about it or other men (and women) will regard him as a poor specimen. It is essential to a man's status amongst his peers that he has laid as many girls as possible, or at least says he has. A man who says 'no' (we are always being reminded that the word still exists) would probably be behaving responsibly but his virile image would slip. The pressures on young boys to perform are as strong as the pressures on young girls not to and both suffer in the process. Boys want sex, not girls: girls want boys, not sex. This is what we call the sex war; this is the land of the seducer and the tease; this is where marriage is offered or withheld.

In 1927 a psychologist wrote: 'A woman by making herself cheap, makes herself nasty; she destroys her own value in the eyes of men. We are so constituted that we value highly only that which costs us much effort and long pursuit. Men will never attach high value to a gratification which they can purchase at a small price or obtain by easy barter.'[2] And in 1972 a trendy psychiatrist advised another generation: 'For the woman who really wants to be sure to marry the man she has chosen, the motto might be, "Promise him anything, but deliver it the night *after* the wedding!" Premarital sex is like gasoline – delivered drop by drop, it provides the power that brings man and woman together. Scattered indiscriminately, it can catch fire and consume any chance for marriage or future happiness.'[3] The tempo differs but it is the same old tune. It might all have some point if it had any basis in reality, but it doesn't. In 1957 figures showed that one in five brides were pregnant by the time they married.

More recent figures show this is now nearer one in ten. We may speculate as to the reasons for the drop (more widespread use of contraception; a more liberal abortion law; fewer shotgun weddings) but the list is unlikely to include an increase in the number of virgin brides.

Many, if not most men now marry women they have slept with before marriage. Many couples now live together until they want children and then marry. It is curious that this behaviour is termed promiscuous rather than immoral, for a woman who shares her home with a man has formed a close relationship and will have little incentive (or opportunity) to sleep around in a casual and promiscuous fashion.

Promiscuity has become a big bogey word; it can be blamed for all social ills and virtually everything encourages it – the pill, liberal abortion, sex education, women's dress. My suspicion that what is really being blamed is the very existence of the female sex was finally confirmed when I read of an hermaphroditic patient in one American clinic who had external genitals which appeared feminine but was found to have no ovaries, uterus or vagina. She naturally wished to have a vagina constructed: 'But her parents opposed this: she was not married at the time, and they felt it would lead to "promiscuity" – although they knew she could not become pregnant since she had neither womb nor ovaries.'[4] The perfect daughter! (To the credit of the medical profession the parents' opposition was overruled.)

It may be acceptable now for women to have sexual feelings but these must only be expressed within marriage. No one has yet explained how self-control is to be maintained by women now that repression is no longer encouraged (though it still operates). The result of all this moralistic conditioning is to make sexual expectations within marriage quite unrealistic. The new permissiveness encourages us to expect fulfilment as a right. The old morality perpetuates attitudes towards sex (filth, obscenity) which create anxiety and inhibit enjoyment. If we really believe that sex is dirty and men are only after one thing, then a wedding ring won't make any difference; our feelings just do not work like that. Nor is it possible to be sexually sophisticated and ecstatically orgasmic with no experience at all. Sexual technique is something we learn by practice and learn best in a relaxed, loving relationship.

Since our attitudes to our sexuality are so desperately confused ('What *is* an orgasm?' women cry, not really trusting their own subjective experience, needing external scientific proof and reassurance), the mother role looks simpler and safer. We are reared to be domestic creatures, told we have an instinct for child care. We copy our mothers' domestic routines, we play with dolls. Of course inanimate plastic dolls with rosebud mouths and long blonde hair (some even have breasts) bear no resemblance to live, wriggling babies. Most young mothers have to be taught how to bath and feed their infants. Even breastfeeding has to be taught. The intimate details of child care are not part of our education but we expect it will all come naturally because we are women.

A situation which focuses our attention exclusively on home and children can produce a fairly logical attitude to marriage and the family which excludes men – your job's done, mate, what matters is me and baby, you just provide the bread and sperm. In one study of adolescent girls' attitudes to work and marriage 600 girls were asked to write an essay on the theme of their imagined future lives. Over a third fantasized the death of their husbands before middle age. Once the men had given them children and the children were past the age of dependence, the men were dispensable.[5]

A sixteen-year-old girl I interviewed had much the same attitude: 'I'd really like a child, I mean that's something I really would want and if I didn't find a man that I wanted to marry or live with for the rest of my life, I'd still have a child.' And later, about childbirth: 'I'd really like my husband to be there, I mean I'd like him to deliver my child if I ever have a child. That's one of my reasons why I'd like to have a husband actually.'

We grow up believing that our fulfilment in life is to marry and have children. If we don't marry we are 'on the shelf', if we do marry but don't have children we are selfish. I have never understood why people who refrain from producing children they don't want and are not prepared to look after should be regarded as selfish. But as far as having children is concerned most women think in terms of when and how many, not whether or not.

Having babies is such a central part of women's role and identity and there is so much pressure to conform to that role or appear unwomanly, that very few of us really think carefully about what we are doing: 'You see other people don't you? You see other people's babies, but then you never really know what that means in terms of twenty-four hours a day. You know, you probably see the nice bits.' Indeed, the situation can become so emotionally loaded that it is impossible to make a rational decision:

A lot of women get in a state where they feel that they want a baby. I mean I'm now twenty-nine and a large pro-portion of my friends who don't have children really have got to the stage where they just want a baby, quite regard-less of whether they have a man they think would be a suitable father. They just want a baby. I think one psycho-logically justifies this, this biological urge by convincing oneself there's something important and fulfilling about having a baby.

I would advise them to think very carefully before they do it, and yet there's this awful dilemma that I think *it's not until you've had a baby that you know whether you really want one or not.* [My italics]

This woman defines the problem very well. We are driven by irrational needs to produce a child without really knowing whether we want to be mothers. The ability to have a child as a proof of womanhood can be so strong that it blots out everything else. This is very common with women who have miscarriages:

I got pregnant and I wasn't the slightest bit bothered about it, it wasn't going to make *any* difference to my life at all and then I had a miscarriage and then I wanted a child like mad after I'd lost it. When I got pregnant the second time, I was quite sure I was going to lose that one as well so I sort of had the impression I was never actually going to be a mother. All through the pregnancy I was absolutely sure it was going to be either backward or mental or something, I wouldn't believe that I was going to be an ordinary mother. And then when he came I still didn't believe it for quite a few weeks, I think because of the miscarriage.

It is common, too, with women who have difficulty conceiving: 'It took me quite a while to get pregnant and because it took me quite a while, the determination to get pregnant was increased.' To *choose* not to have children and to be *unable* to have children are two very different situations, comparable to the difference between a celibate and an impotent man. The ability to conceive, carry and give birth to a baby is an important part of a woman's sexual identity, and failure can be felt as a desperate loss. Childbearing, however, is a very different matter to child rearing and in the urgent desire to prove ourselves 'real women', the fact is easily overlooked.

Even when the reasons for wanting a baby seem to be fairly straightforward, there can be hidden motives:

We always knew we wanted kids, it was almost an unspoken thing, and I got to the state where I felt I would like to have a baby. Now, it was just literally as simple as that but looking back on it I realize that in fact I wanted a baby for all sorts of reasons, the main one being that I'd got to the stage with my job where I knew I'd been there too long and I knew I had to leave but I couldn't tear myself away. Looking back on it having a baby was both a let out from that particular situation and from the work situation in general.

This woman's experience is remarkably common. Women often choose to have a baby as a way of escaping from a difficult or boring work situation. Instead of trying to solve the work problems, or find a different job, as a man would have to do, women turn to motherhood as an attractive alternative. It looks like an easy option. It isn't. To have a baby in order to escape from work can be rather like jumping from the frying pan into an inferno; the monotony, drudgery, low status and isolation of motherhood are delivered to us with the baby.

In one study of the attitude of working-class schoolgirls, it was discovered that the majority were pleased they were destined to be wives and mothers instead of being committed to the social evil of having to do a job for the rest of their lives.[6] In another study, *The Captive Wife*, Hannah Gavron comments that though the working-class wives in her sample seemed to accept their roles as wives and mothers more readily in theory, in fact they were psychologically unprepared for the results. The impact of motherhood on middle-class wives was felt especially as a loss of independence. Ninety-two per cent of middle-class mothers and eighty-seven per cent of working-class mothers intended to return to work.[7]

So motives for having a baby can be confused, even with accidents:

I had an accident, sort of an accident, it wasn't exactly an accident because we knew that we had the chance of having a kid and in fact we even mentioned it; I mean I wasn't married. It was a really difficult situation in fact and it was very funny finding I was pregnant, I was very happy in a way. I think I wanted to have children before I met his dad. I think that was partly why I got together with his dad. In a funny kind of way it was sort of almost like a biological thing. I was feeling broody, you know, friends had babies and I was seeing them with them. I don't know whether I just wanted to escape out of the world of work or something.

It can seem as though a child might give meaning to life when other things have failed:

I think to be really honest it was because I hadn't found any satisfaction in anything else and I believed I'd make a very good mother. With me it was a fundamental need to have a child because I'm a very lazy person, I'm extremely lazy and I needed something to do. I sat on my backside for years and I needed something as important as a human being to take on my time, to *demand* my time, to make me realize how precious time was. So it was pretty selfish really.

To expect a child to provide this kind of fulfilment places a very heavy burden on the child. We should not expect our children to provide us with a meaning in life, though we are encouraged to. We should not expect them to provide us with love and the security of being needed. It is we who should be providing love and security for them. The false expectation that children will satisfy our emotional needs can lead to great unhappiness. In her book on baby battering, *Children in Danger*, Jean Renvoize discusses the kind of attitudes typical of battering parents:

> Together with this insistence on absolute obedience usually goes a pathetic demand for clearly expressed love. The parents want what they never had in their own infancy – uncritical love – and who better than their own children to give it to them? Unfortunately they do not realize that small children are very self-occupied creatures: infants need to pass through many stages of development before they are ready to offer selfless love to anybody.[8]

Nor need we see such parents as a poor sad few; they exist as one end of a continuing scale. I wonder how many of us always remember that a screaming baby is demanding love and care, not, as we so often feel, rejecting it – and us.

So, when she is confronted with pregnancy, a woman not only has to deal with the physical changes within her body, she also has to come to terms with cultural and personal assumptions of which previously she may have been blithely unaware. Her adjustment to childbearing will depend on her expectations of herself as a mother and her ability to adapt the role to her own needs.

Dana Breen, a psychologist, concludes from her research on women well-adjusted to motherhood:

> Those women who are most adjusted to childbearing are those who are less enslaved by the experience, have more

differentiated, more open appraisals of themselves and other people, do not aspire to be the perfect selfless mother which they might have felt their own mother had not been but are able to call on a good mother image with which they can identify, and do not experience themselves as passive, the cultural stereotype of femininity.[9]

When we give birth we cross an invisible dividing line. We may fight this feeling or try to ignore it, but in the end it has to be faced. The act of pushing a baby into the world does not make us different people but that new life alters all the relationships around us and everyone has to adjust.

The extent to which we can make our adjustment will depend on more than how quickly our hormones get back to normal. The amount of emotional support we receive is important as are the ways in which we find it possible to combine the monotony and isolation of the housewife's life with the joy and fascination of a relationship with a fast-developing human being, our child.

Expectations of motherhood in our society are over-romantic and unrealistic. It is talked of in glowing terms, but in the status game it is way down at the bottom of the league. If we seriously believe that we are going to get any thanks or recognition for our work as mothers, we are in for a nasty shock. If we do the job adequately, it is taken for granted that it is 'natural' to us, if we do it badly we will be castigated by just about everyone in sight. It is a cast iron guarantee that the more motherhood is idealized, the more women are enslaved by it.

Since the mother receives little social esteem, her reward has to come from the child. It must be bright, clean, smart, well-behaved and loving for it is her handiwork, her reflection. If the child fails to live up to expectations it may be neglected, over-protected, or in some cases actually battered. We have all been fucked up in one way or another by our mothers, poor souls, and I am afraid it will continue happening until society starts valuing the job mothers do and makes their working conditions more tolerable.

Experts in child psychology agree that a mother who does

not love herself cannot love her child; that a mother who is unhappy and frustrated cannot respond to the needs of her child. Children reflect the emotional state of their mothers and they recognize pretence and insincerity. Advice aimed at altering maternal behaviour without taking account of the mother's needs and emotions is doomed to failure. Yet it pours out. Most of it is based on the ideal of the eternally self-sacrificing mother; an ideal which is more romantic than realistic and helpful to neither mother nor child.

The ultimate entry into womanhood, the punishment for sexuality, the price of motherhood is the famous pain of childbirth.

> A woman's life is all in vain
> Three minutes pleasure
> Nine months pain
> Three weeks rest and at it again
> A woman's life is all in vain.

I learnt that merry little jingle at my good Methodist boarding school from some enlightened contemporary. It reflects the curse of Eve – 'In sorrow shalt thou bring forth children' – and the anger of women in maternity wards – 'Bloody men, if they had babies there'd only be one in each family.' Childbirth is a woman's reproductive burden and her destiny. The fact that this no longer need be the case is altering attitudes to labour only very slowly.

Expectations of childbirth range from the belief that it will be a positive achievement and a major life experience, to the fear that it will be agony and a real trial by fire. The reality is that labours are as different as the babies they produce. Nature is indiscriminate and works according to her own laws without regard to justice or compassion. We can interfere with those laws or learn to control them to our own benefit, as we do with contraception, but we cannot alter the laws themselves.

The experience of pain is notoriously subjective. Men and women can withstand appalling torture to protect their comrades. Women can come through long and difficult labours with little memory of pain. I personally doubt whether pain-less childbirth exists without anaesthetic. It is more a matter of how it is experienced on the continuum between discomfort and agony. Frequently the pain is experienced as unbearable because the woman is afraid, ignorant and *alone*. Education in the processes and sensations of pregnancy and labour can help us to feel actively in control of what is happening, not just a passive body being delivered. As Dana Breen's research shows, this sense of activity is important if we are to adjust well to motherhood. Antenatal classes are available but there are not enough good ones. Many hospitals and clinics run their own classes but these are often very sketchy and not al-ways reassuring ('they talked about the pain that every woman must go through to have a baby'). There is no *must* about pain in childbirth; pain is an experience and cannot be measured objectively. This does not mean that pain is psycho-logical, imaginary or self-induced, but that it is only the woman herself who knows what she is experiencing and how well she can cope with it.

Whatever the reality when it comes, childbirth education for the non-pregnant barely exists. Few girls in our society have close contact with pregnant women or small babies. If an older sister or an aunt is pregnant it will be watched with curiosity but questions are rarely asked because it is all associated with sex and pain and is a generally embarrassing topic.

Then there is the vagina to consider. The vagina is the birth passage. All of us not delivered by Caesarean section travelled down our mother's vagina to greet the world. It is marvellously soft and elastic, stretching to ease the baby out into the world without damage. It is also, of course, the place where penetration occurs during intercourse and it is because of this sexual function that women regard it with shame. In *The Female Eunuch* Germaine Greer concludes her chapter on cunt hatred by saying: 'Women are reputed never to be disgusted. The sad fact is that they often are, but not with men; following the lead of men, they are most often disgusted with themselves.'[10] And I believe that for a large number of women this is true. As young girls we know very little about our vaginas; our mothers rarely give it a name and few of us dare to use a mirror to look at it. Little boys usually grow up with a pet name for their penis, willie or winkie or somesuch. Little girls have to make do with their 'bottom' which totally ignores the fact that the vagina exists as a separate and important piece of their anatomy.

'The first month I was at college some of my friends were twittering about a girl down the hall. She was having a painful time trying to learn to put in a tampon. Finally someone helped her and found she was trying to put it into her anus.'[11] This kind of ignorance is bound to create feelings of anxiety which masquerade as modesty. One woman I talked to said she was desperately worried about the painful stitches following her episiotomy (the cut made to ease delivery) but could not face using a mirror to look at them. She preferred to wait and ask the doctor at her postnatal examination. She would not have reacted in the same way if she had had a sore throat. I must admit that I had a little more courage when worried for the same reason, but it came as a real moment of truth to discover that I felt intensely embarrassed squatting over a mirror in the privacy of a locked bathroom to see why I hurt. It takes more than intellectual understanding to uproot inhibitions.

Because women feel so anxious and insecure about their vaginas, internal examinations can be a real nightmare, particularly if the doctor is insensitive, as many are. An internal examination always has sexual connotations. It is felt as an invasion of privacy and especially embarrassing when performed by a male doctor. Being examined by a woman is a less sexually loaded situation and it would be nice to believe that women doctors were more considerate, but unfortunately it is not always true. It often seems as though female medical students have to outmen the men in order to succeed at all. This is not universally true and it is to be hoped that as more women enter medical schools the trait will disappear.

Since the vagina is never talked about, children frequently believe that babies are sicked up, arrive from women's bottoms or somehow through the tummy. I believed for many years that your tummy started splitting open and that's why it hurt and you needed a doctor. Women who have had babies rarely discuss the experience with those who haven't. There seems to be a sort of taboo and sense of initiation about the whole thing; it is women's business, not for young girls.

In part this reticence springs from the connection between birth, sex and the vagina, topics which older women find it difficult to discuss with the young. It also springs from the general air of mystery surrounding the female reproductive system with its hidden passages and monthly cycles. Experiencing the pain of childbirth is also undoubtedly a passport to womanhood. In their fascinating study *Patterns of Infant Care in an Urban Community* the Newsons comment:

In our society, as in many others, the birth of a first child is more than a biological event. It carries overtones of a ceremonial rite whereby a young woman is initiated into the established matriarchy. Like the acquisition of a wedding ring, the bearing of the first (legitimate) child confers enhanced status. And, as with most rites of passage, whether they concern a tribal initiation into manhood or an English boy's admission to his public school peer group, the prestige of the initiated is maintained by the tradition of ordeal by pain and suffering: a slowly changing tradition.[12]

Childbirth is what separates the women from the girls, though I cannot agree that the birth of a first child any longer confers enhanced status. This, of course, is part of the problem. I was certainly disconcerted after the remarkably easy birth of my first daughter, Imogen, to discover that I was ostracized in the maternity ward. 'You wouldn't know about it,' other patients said. The implication was that it hadn't hurt enough and I was therefore disqualified as a full-blooded initiate. In a sense, of course, it is always annoying to see that others achieve easily what we struggle and suffer to obtain, be it a job, a house or a baby. The dismissive attitude towards those women who have had an easy labour, however, seems to me to be more than anger at life's injustices. Childbirth *should* be painful and the more you suffer the more of a woman you are. These attitudes are slowly changing, particularly with the increased use of epidurals (local anaesthetic injected into the spine) which can guarantee pain-free labour (though they increase the likelihood of a forceps delivery). The problem with using drugs to remove pain is that they remove all other sensations as well and they also affect the baby.

But, despite all the fear about childbirth, at least there will be the baby to love at the end of it all. The widespread belief in maternal instinct leads women to expect that marvellous, radiant mother-love will suddenly arrive as the baby is born. But many women feel nothing for their babies until days and sometimes months after the birth. This is a common reaction, especially after a drugged birth. Giving birth can be very tiring and the baby is a stranger, as yet an unknown quantity. It is only our society's insistence that all maternal feelings must be positive which makes women feel guilty about an initial indifference. This story is fairly typical:

I wasn't terribly interested in the baby, particularly so because you know they give you the baby to carry upstairs before they've washed it and there was this peculiar, still vaguely bloodstained creature that I had in my arms and I thought he looked absolutely hideous. And then I got up to the ward about seven, I was given something to eat and then the doctor came to say that there was some trouble with Andrew's breathing. They hadn't got all the mucus out of his lungs or whatever it is and they were going to put him in an incubator for the night. That absolutely terrified me, I mean, I said to the doctor, 'Is he going to be all right?' and you know what doctors are like, they won't say yes, they say 'Well we see no reason why not but I would like to have him in an incubator so I can monitor his heart' and all this sort of thing. So I was fairly convinced he was going to die, so I thought, well what's the point in being interested because he's probably going to die anyway.

Clearly this mother's initial feeling of indifference was not helped by the way in which her fears for the baby's health were treated. In this kind of situation women may either become frantic with worry or, as in this case, simply switch off.

Mother-baby bonding (the relationship formed between mother and baby at birth) is the subject of much concern. As long as the child-rearing role continues to be the major responsibility of the biological mother in our society this bonding is essential to the baby's future growth and happiness. If the rush of mother-love fails to appear, we feel guilty and anxious, and in this situation a hospital atmosphere does not help.

> The woman in hospital cannot fight for what she thinks is right (for example keeping the baby with her); she is in too novel a situation to know if she should object to instructions given to her on the right procedures to use with the baby. There is also, in hospitals, a taboo against expressing meaningful feelings. It is all right to be angry or 'weep' for nothing as a result of your hormones but not to have feelings about hospital procedures or feelings about the baby which are not positive (these too must be 'sterilized' like the bottles).[13]

When things go wrong it can affect a vital relationship at its root. Many women I have talked to have suggested that perhaps their behaviour towards one particular child (usually the most 'difficult') had been affected by a bad birth experience. John Bowlby in his famous study of maternal deprivation writes:

> Let the reader reflect on the astonishing practice which has been followed in maternity wards – of separating mothers and babies immediately after birth – and ask himself whether this is the way to promote a close mother-child relationship. It is hoped that this madness of Western society will never be copied by the so-called less developed countries![14]

Well, perhaps if babies were delivered by psychiatrists instead of obstetricians there might be a little more sanity. As it is, the different specialities within medicine appear to take very little notice of each other until public opinion compels them to do so.

There are obviously a number of factors which affect the way a mother feels about her baby at birth and it would be simplistic to suggest that the birth experience is the only or even the major one. It is an area which has been ignored for too long, however, and I shall be dealing with it more fully in later chapters.

When I was depressed after the birth of my second child, Pippa, a woman said to me, 'What do you do with your natural resentment towards the children?' – *natural!* Isn't it wrong and unnatural to resent the tiny baby who never asked to be born and is totally dependent on you? I think we feel it is, but resentment exists and needs to be expressed. It is acknowledged that mothers of battered babies can be helped enormously simply by discussing their problems with each other in the knowledge that they will not be condemned. Baby battering is an extreme example of what can happen when resentment builds up without being allowed meaningful expression.

Sometimes we blame ourselves and feel guilty, inadequate and worthless; sometimes we over-protect the baby, feeling it is in some way threatened; sometimes we turn on our husband; lousy sod, it's a man's world all right!

One of the most common misconceptions is that children will cement a marriage. They may well block available escape routes for a time but they certainly will not revitalize a bad relationship. In America a study of 800 couples by Dr Harold Feldman at Cornell University showed there were significantly lower levels of marital happiness among couples with children.[15] A sad comment about the traditionally happy event and a reflection on the way in which society fails to integrate parents and children. One experienced marriage counsellor has written: 'Instead of strengthening a poor marriage, the arrival of a baby could bring it finally to the divorce court – and it is sad to note that the greatest number of divorces do occur after the birth of the first child.'[16]

The stresses which affect the wife are bound to affect the husband, and men are understandably upset when the mother-lover conflict starts taking its toll of their wives' sexual responses; and perhaps it influences their own appetite more than they would care to admit.

> If the wife is breastfeeding it interferes because between you and her are those two bloody great breasts full of milk and there is a sort of taboo about the milk. It is not unpleasant in itself to taste but it has rather repulsive connotations insofar as it is rather like in a way sleeping with your mother. The breasts don't belong to you, they belong to the baby.

That is the comment of one remarkably honest young father. In her book *The Baby Trap* Ellen Peck quotes the opinion of a Freudian psychiatrist: 'Well, the men can complain about *lack of responsiveness* all they want. It's somewhat of a cop-out to say that. It's really a matter also of lack of attraction to the wife, once she becomes a mother. A man's sexual response to the mother figure – well, let's say it's often ambivalent at best.'[17] Whatever a man's problems (and I deal with these in a separate chapter) he never experiences the complete upheaval of every area of his life which a new mother experiences. She must adjust to a completely new way of life which is disarmingly familiar; she is now the mother in a domestic situation which she associates with childhood. Domesticity is familiar to us all as children but being a mother is very different. The mother is restricted physically and mentally, tied to the needs of a totally helpless and dependent infant whom she both loves and resents. She also has to cope with the reality of endless chores and shapeless days, usually spent in isolation.

Her husband may expect her to be the same bright, carefree girl she used to be, or she may feel that he does. Her first commitment, however, must be to love and care for her baby, husband and home. If love fails and life is not the bed of roses it is supposed to be, then she has failed, and is less than a woman, as well as being trapped. It is within this plethora of confused expectations that postnatal depression blooms, a black rose.

2. *Ann's Story*

You may find yourself crying bitterly without any real reason for it. This happens to many women and is of *no importance* so don't worry about it. [My italics]

> BMA publication, *You and Your Baby*, given free by hospitals to expectant mothers.

'When I got home I was in a state of complete trance. I got home with the baby and it all seemed terribly enormous to me, you know? I didn't know what had hit me. Of course now I realize it was this damned depression.

'I got home. Pete's father was here. He seemed too much. He was all over me because it was my birthday the day I got home. There were flowers and there were cards. I knew I had to say "Thank you" but I couldn't get it out. I just didn't have the mental strength to say "Thank you" to show that I was pleased.

'I wandered round with the baby in my arms from one room to the other, looking at the place. I couldn't put him down, it was sort of like a magnet. I couldn't put him down at all. Pete finally took him out of my arms and put him in the pram. I sat around dazed.

'I felt as though I'd been in isolation for several months. I looked out of the window and I saw all these people going past and I thought, "There's people! There's people outside!" I felt there'd been a complete break in my life. It was almost as though I'd been, not a very kind comparison, but as if I'd been in prison, you know? It took a hell of a lot of getting used to.

'The next day I felt ecstatically happy. I asked Pete to buy this record I'd heard on the radio and I got overcome with sentimentality which I hate in me. I found myself dancing to it in the bathroom and every time I turned it up the baby went quiet because he cried a lot. I thought "Ahhhh Tom's record", sort of thing and that was the only time I felt happy for ten weeks! The first and only time, well, I was obviously sort of high at the time.

'Then things just got worse and worse. Somehow the slightest thing made me burst into tears. Pete would find me holding the baby, holding him to me with my head bowed and tears pelting down my face. He'd come in and say, "What is it? What's the matter?" I could see he felt helpless and . . . somehow I wanted him to help me; yet I didn't know what I wanted. So I just sat there with helpless tears, he stood there looking confused and utterly bored. His very confusion made me feel everything was even more futile. It just got desperate.

'Everything . . . I don't know whether one can feel futile but everything seemed futile, you know. Nothing I did seemed to please the baby for a start. I felt helpless. It seemed like a project that I just couldn't get to the end of, I couldn't achieve anything. Every single thing that I did, he bawled his head off at, he never smiled, was never happy. You don't expect them to smile at that age, but he never seemed satisfied.

'I didn't blame myself really, I just was terribly worried that he was unhappy. He seemed so desperate and then somehow I found myself getting more and more miserable. It wasn't because he was unhappy, I know that, it was just *me*, you know? Because he was unhappy it made it worse. And I went into a black pit.

'For a start not a single thought went past my head. Nothing. Total blank, absolute blank. Because I remember sitting in a heap and I must have probably had my mouth open. I felt absolutely gormless. I was feeding this baby in a trance. Pete was looking at me very confused and I thought, "I wonder what I look like" – so I must have had one thought! It was as though I was totally incapable of handling anything I did. Everything I was doing I was doing automatically, I had no mastery over it. I had no control over it at all.

'After three weeks I went out of the flat. I couldn't leave the baby; I was terrified of leaving the baby. I don't know why, I was just terrified of leaving the baby. I took him out in the pram. I was walking and I crossed the street as though he wasn't in front of me. Because I remember, it was fascinating, fascinating to watch the cars go by so close to the pram. I just didn't have control over it. I saw it happening as if I wasn't there. Instinct must have made me draw the pram back because he's still with me, but I remember watching it, fascinated. They must have gone by by centimetres.

'Everything I did was like that, it must have been because I had no control over myself. It was lethargy and a complete disorientation from my own body. I was watching my body do things.

'I thought perhaps it was the breastfeeding . . . I remember this awful feeling every time the baby cried and the milk came into my body. It hurt, it hurt like hell. As the milk came, the tears came and as the tears came I felt incapable of anything. In fact I can feel it so acutely now, I can remember that feeling. I think I resented that terrific physical hold he had over me; that I had to be there, me, physically, had to be there. And even then he wasn't happy when I was there, so it was compounded. It was like digging earth upon earth; everything got harder underneath.

'It never entered my head to ask for help. Nothing entered my head. The welfare officer came round three or four times and the health visitor came round more frequently. They might have noticed something but they certainly didn't tell me and they asked if I was all right. "Are you all right in yourself?" and I remember saying, "Well, my breasts aren't hurting me." I thought in physical terms immediately, but no, I was all right, physically, fine thank you very much.

'It went on for ten weeks. I slowly began to realize that something was wrong, so something must have started to work again. I slowly began to realize this wasn't the normal me. I *couldn't* understand why he was crying so much, why I felt so awfully disorientated, why I had no energy for anything. I knew I was terribly tired, that was only to be expected.

'I remember thinking, "If only somebody would take the baby off my hands for forty-eight hours, I'm sure I'd be able to cope. If I could sleep for forty-eight hours. If I just

didn't have anything to do with the baby for forty-eight . . ."
I remember that forty-eight hours ringing through my head
you know . . . I felt so responsible for him, I felt I wasn't able
to cope, I wasn't able to help him until I regained my own
strength, mental and physical. Well, mental didn't enter my
head, I thought it was my physical body. It never entered my
head there was anything wrong with my mind, I thought it
was my body that needed a rest.

'One day I begged my mother to come over because Pete
had gone out. I started crying and I thought, "This is daft,
there's something very wrong with me." Funnily enough, I
think I was probably on the mend when I realized that. My
mother came over and I just let it roll out in floods and it's
not as though I could put my finger on anything. I don't
know what I must have said to her. She didn't know what I
was talking about in the sense that she hadn't had anything
like that after I was born, but she had very recently been
through a very severe depression. She said that everything
I was talking about was a case of severe depression.

'Having talked about it gave a certain ring of sanity to it all
There was something to grip on to there. Somebody had had
the same as I had, somebody knew what I was talking about.
I was so pleased to have it identified; the relief of knowing
what it was, it was incredible. It was like the floodgates
opening. At last I knew, I could hang on to something definite
then.

'Very slowly I started feeling better. I found I was able
to do things . . . good thoughts in my head. One day I actually had a whole range of wonderful, mundane thoughts . . .
it was exciting. I think that second to having Tom, that's
the most exciting experience of my life, just to have all the
very dull thoughts go through my head. I believed I was on
the mend. Looking back on it I must have been a long time
on the mend because I've only just started to relax. I know
that because I'm very taut across the shoulders, everything's
very taut, and that's me when I'm nervy.

'I've tried to think of what it could have been, I mean, you
hear that it's hormones. All I know is that I was happy with
that baby when he was born. I was really excited about it.

I just wanted to show that child I was going to have every-thing that I'd found exciting and interesting in this world.

'The terrific heaviness over my head lifted at about ten weeks but as I say, looking back on it, I think I've only just started to get back to normal, and he's six months old now.'

3. On the Road

Few women know that depression is the most common complication of the period following childbirth. Few women are forewarned when they are pregnant or observed carefully after delivery. At a time when we are under intensive medical care, one in ten of us (the number is probably higher than that) will find ourselves depressed, confused and unsupported.

Postnatal depression falls between medical specialities and gets lost. Obstetricians do not consider it has anything to do with them. Psychiatrists do not work in maternity hospitals and anyway do not consider that depression following childbirth is any different from depression occurring at other times. (Official statistics do not give separate figures for postnatal depression. It is lumped together with depression occurring at other times of life.) But the fact is that a large proportion of cases of depression in the community occur after the birth of a baby.

One study which summarizes thirty-seven reports published from all parts of the world shows that with the exception of a few developing countries in Africa and India, twice as many women as men become depressed.[1] Another study of referred mental illnesses in Chichester and Salisbury found the highest referral rates to local psychiatric services for neurotic and reactive depressions were among married women aged twenty-five to thirty-four: this is also the peak age for having children (in the 1971 census 51 per cent of married women in this age group had a child under five).[2] Yet another study of 2257 women who had a child in 1970 using the Camberwell psychiatric register found that the new episode rate for psychosis and depressive illness rose sharply in women in the first three months after delivery. There was a less dramatic but more sustained rise from the tenth month.[3]

All these studies deal with referred (i.e. treated) cases of depression but together what they show is that women suffer from depression more than men; women who suffer most from depression have a child under five; of women with children the greatest time of risk is in the first three months after delivery. Postnatal depression is therefore a particular and specific problem. It has received little attention:

> What lies between the extremes of severe puerperal depression, with the risks of suicide and, perhaps, infanticide, occurring after no more than 1 in 500 births, on the one hand, and the trivial weepiness of 'the Blues', said to follow up to 80 per cent of deliveries on the other? The frequent occurrence of states of depression post-partum much less dramatic than the former, yet decidedly more disabling than the latter, is perhaps fairly generally known, but has received little investigation.

So writes Brice Pitt, one of the few people to have studied the problem. His research with a random sample of 305 pregnant women showed that thirty-three (10.8%) were suffering from depression six to eight weeks following delivery and a further nineteen (6.2%) were doubtfully depressed.

A year later twelve of the depressed group (43%) had not improved. Only five of the thirty-three depressed women were receiving treatment at the time of the study and only two of the twelve who had not improved after a year received any treatment.[4]

If the birth rate in Britain is somewhere in the region of 550,000 a year this means that about 60,500 women, at least, suffer from postnatal depression each year with 26,000 being handicapped for more than a year.

In the course of researching this book I have been asked many times what causes postnatal depression and what I felt caused mine. There are two main theories about the causes. One is a physical explanation about adjustment to hormone levels which I consider fully in Chapter 15. The other has been summarized by Dr Desmond Bardon, consultant psychiatrist at Shenley Hospital, Hertfordshire, as 'stress acting on predisposition'.[5] This latter view is supported by a recent study of the social origins of depression by George Brown, Professor of Sociology at Bedford College, London, and his colleague Tirril Harris. They found that depression, in most cases, was caused by stressful 'life events' such as bereavement, separation, moving house or husband's unemployment (loss situations) or by major hardships, such as bad housing, which continue for at least two years.

There were four vulnerability factors which predispose women to depression in these circumstances though they do not cause depression on their own. These factors are: lack of a close and confidential relationship; loss of their mother before the age of eleven either through death or separation; having three or more children under fourteen living at home; and the lack of an outside job. The feature all these have in common is that they lower self-esteem.[6]

Since almost all newly delivered mothers lack an outside job we are all, by definition, 25 per cent predisposed to depression. In addition, having a baby is a stressful 'life event' in its own right so we are all dealing with one stress. It is not hard to see in this context how all women are to some extent vulnerable to depression following birth.

After we have given birth it is as if we wake up to discover that a mountain of sand has been deposited in front of the doors of our home. Some women get to work energetically to dig routes out. They have friends who come along and help. They work round the sand and over the sand; they find marvellously inventive ways to cope with the situation. Some women find one difficult route out and stick to that. Some try to dig a way through and get buried, others just look at it, feel defeated, retreat within their four walls and give up.

Psychologists concern themselves with the reasons why some of us can be energetic and find routes out and others get buried or trapped. The latter are often called 'inadequate personalities' and ways to help them are suggested. This ignores the essential question of why the sand need be there in the first place. For the sand represents the ways in which the new mother is isolated from the outside world. This has little to do with her personal psychology. It is a matter of social organization and social attitudes. 'At present women are being blamed for being unhappy about a life situation which they did not create and which they cannot control and they are labelled as neurotic when they attempt to articulate the

confusion and directionless dimensions of that situation.'[7]
This comment sums up very well the kind of situation in
which the new mother finds herself.

I am discussing the subject of postnatal depression therefore within the framework of what I consider to be a hostile
environment for all new mothers. Childbirth and the postnatal
period are situations of stress anyway but in our society the
stress is far more extreme than it needs to be.

I see the picture of a depression like a stained glass window with varying sized fragments of different-coloured
glass joined together by lead. The windows all show a picture
of mother and child and all must conform to a standard shape
and size. It is the formation of the total image which differs
with each woman, the way in which the fragments are soldered
together to make an individual pattern. I now want to examine
some of the fragments, see what kind of experiences fit, like
the coloured glass, into the framework we are all given. One of
the major emotional stresses is the experience of birth
itself.

Are pregnancy and childbirth normal, natural events or are
they a medical illness? Incredibly, American courts of law
have sat in judgement on this issue and found in favour of
the medical definition.

In most states of America midwifery is illegal. Norman
Casserley, practising as a lay midwife in California (where
midwives are legal only if they carry a certificate that does
not exist!), was prosecuted for practising medicine without a
licence: 'At his trial in March 1972, Norman based his defence on the premise that the practice of midwifery
has nothing to do with the practice of medicine or any
of its functions of diagnosis, medication or surgery, and that
pregnancy is neither a sickness nor an abnormal condition.
He was convicted on three counts of practising without a
licence.'[8]

Again in California, following a police raid on the Santa
Cruz Birth Center, lay midwives working there were prosecuted in the same way and used the same defence: 'In an
initial ruling earlier in the spring the district court of appeals
held that the women could not be charged with a crime, stat-

ing that childbirth is not an illness, deformity or disease, and that therefore midwifery does not constitute the practice of medicine. Just two months later, the same three judges granted a re-hearing on the case and reversed their decision.'[9]

The struggle between the Californian midwives and the massed powers of the medical establishment is one which is taking place against a background of consumer demand for home births. Some American women are so concerned about the high technology overkill in American maternity hospitals that they believe that it is not only more satisfying but physically safer for them to have their babies at home. American doctors, like good businessmen, do not want to lose trade. They are therefore acting to preserve their monopoly. One way of doing this is to claim that birth is a medical emergency.

Well, thank God for the National Health Service! But can we afford to be so smug? Certainly midwifery has always been legal in Britain and our consultants have only a limited area in which to work for profit. It is, however, the policy of the government to encourage 100 per cent hospital confinements and the high technology which so concerns American women is now widespread in our own hospitals. Our courts of law may not have declared pregnancy and birth to be medical illnesses but many of our obstetricians are acting as though they were.

Doctors are trained to think in terms of sickness, not health. In medical terms health is the absence of symptoms. Health is not studied, only pathology. Medical and psychological research concerns itself with the abnormal; healthy, well-adjusted, confident people are not the concern of medicine. Obstetricians are trained to detect and, if possible, correct complications which may occur during pregnancy and labour. Because they know all the things that can go wrong, it is their job to suspect every uterus they examine of not functioning properly until proved otherwise. In antenatal care the advantages of this approach are overwhelming: 'When women have no antenatal care at all, the perinatal mortality rate (that is the death of the baby in the last weeks of pregnancy, at birth, or within the first week after) shoots up by an incredible 500 per cent.'[10] In labour they are less obvious. If her pregnancy has been perfectly normal does a woman need the sort of intensive care hospitals provide for sick people? Is she sick?

One specialist in community medicine, writing about induction as a part of 'office-hour obstetrics' has said:

> The argument from the staff point of view was that there would always be a highly qualified member of staff present if the hospital was on a nine-to-five day week. Whether this was acceptable depended on whether the public accepted that all childbirth was abnormal and should be under a consultant in hospital or whether it could be counted as a normal function.[11]

I hope it will never become acceptable to consider childbirth as an abnormal function. The very proposition is anti-feminist for if it is abnormal to bear children, it is abnormal to be female:

> Parallel to Freud's conception of the male as the proto- type of the human being with the female seen as an in- complete man, there has been a tendency to consider specifically female states as illnesses. Menstruation, preg- nancy, menopause are often construed as illnesses and women are encouraged to consider them as such. To equate these states with illness is dangerous and prevents a real understanding of women.[12]

This tendency to consider specifically female states as ill- nesses perhaps comes naturally to a male-dominated pro- fession. The female reproductive system must seem strange to any man; the trouble starts when that sense of strangeness is communicated to women as fact. Hospitals being associ- ated with sickness, it is all too easy for this to happen. The enormous expansion in convenience induction of labour and increased technological interference in the course of normal labour reflects this tendency to see labour as an abnormal condition. If the purpose of the maternity unit is to ensure live births and the act of birth is regarded as potentially dangerous for the baby, then the logical course of action is to get the baby out as quickly as possible by any appropriate means.

The effectiveness of these methods has been challenged because they are medically unproven and may, in some cases, be damaging. I challenge them for different reasons. I question the assumptions which lead obstetricians to advise women not to trust their bodies. Are we just not up to the job of giving birth? Can the obstetricians do it better? This is clearly not a medical point but a political one. Those doctors who argue that if we accept medical care at the beginning of pregnancy we should accept medical control throughout are, in fact, claiming all birth as a medical emergency.

This is the arrogance of medical science which was once the art of medicine. Obstetrics is becoming all uterus and no womb; clinical, mechanistic, objective principles now control instead of aiding the natural, creative act. The mother is getting far more help than she asked for and her body which nurtured and protected her baby is being seen as threatening and dangerous. Once doctors regard birth simply as a technical process, they become vets handling valuable livestock and deny all human culture.

The problem with hospitalized childbirth lies in this area of clinical versus subjective experience. Some hospitals manage to bring the two together in harmony but not very many. The depersonalized and dehumanized atmosphere in hospitals is not restricted to maternity wards though, obviously, that is what concerns me most in this book. Hospitals are large, cost-conscious institutions where both staff and patients are caught up in a productive system fitting in with resource and time schedules. Sometimes it is fondly imagined that the hospital exists to benefit the patient; to a certain extent it does, but the patient must bend to the hospital for the hospital will not adapt to the patient. The efficiency of the maternity unit is measured in live births, not in happy mothers. Both should be essential aims.

Thus the newly pregnant woman may believe that she is involved in a perfectly normal process which her body is properly equipped to perform and no doctor will directly disabuse her of this notion. She will, however, discover that she is treated as though she were involved in a very dangerous undertaking. She will be told that it is unsafe to have her baby outside a fully equipped hospital, and having gone into that system she is likely to emerge having been treated with drips and drugs, attached to electronic machines, cut and stitched and generally feeling that the whole thing has been like an operation. This is frightening. It is de-humanizing. Fear causes stress which contributes to depres-sion. Loss of dignity leads to a loss of self-esteem, a de-pressed state. The way we experience birth affects the way we experience ourselves as women and as mothers:

> I had an internal examination at the hospital just before she was due, and the examination ruptured the membrane. I leaked for a week without realizing it. When it was finally spotted I was induced. I know the hospital was under-staffed and very busy, but the whole thing was disastrous.
>
> The drip was not regulated properly, and I was in inter-mediate labour, the really painful bit, for hours. Finally they injected me for a forceps delivery, then decided I needed a Caesarean operation quickly.
>
> Because I had her under an operation, I wasn't sure she was mine when I was finally handed her. I can't help wondering if I hadn't been examined so late, I would have given birth naturally. I feel bitter about it.
>
> I was depressed for eighteen months after the birth. I've changed a lot since I had her. I don't think I'll ever be the same again.[18]

It is not uncommon for Caesarean operations to be per-formed because an induction fails (I shall consider induction in Chapter 5). What this woman's story clearly indicates is that *she* connects a long postnatal depression directly with a bad birth experience which she feels was a doctor-created emergency. She wanted to give birth naturally and had lost that experience. Her labour had been artificially controlled throughout.

Because birth has come to be seen as a medical condition requiring treatment by doctors in hospitals, women are there-fore giving birth in an unfamiliar, often frightening environment. They are frequently left alone for long periods of time whilst in labour. They are separated from family, friends and younger children. They share the most private and personal of all experiences with strangers. Margaret Mead has said of birth: 'No primitive society leaves the mother alone, nor does any leave her alone among strangers.'[14] It has taken modern civilization to encourage such a thing.

4. *First Steps in Alienation*

It is men who decide how, where and, increasingly, when women will give birth. This is a situation which inevitably creates alienation. It is not simply that it is difficult for male obstetricians to understand the emotions and sensations of pregnancy and birth. Usually they just do not want to understand; they don't feel it is their business to understand.

Towards the end of my first pregnancy I attended a lecture given by an obstetrician at the hospital where I was to have my baby. He talked to a group of some thirty pregnant women about the development of the foetus and the onset of labour. At the end of the talk one woman asked him if contractions felt anything like period pains. 'I don't know,' he said, 'I haven't had either.' Had he been asked if small-pox was anything like chickenpox and given that reply we might have been forgiven for questioning his competence.

Obstetrics must be one of the only areas of medicine where the sensations experienced by the patient are not regarded as significant. So many women are told they 'can't be' ready to push and end up delivering their babies in the wrong place:

I was in the ward and they kept asking me if I was having pains yet, and I said I had them in my legs, in my thighs, which is where I do get them. They said, 'Nonsense, you don't have them in your legs.' I said, 'Well, I do.' But they took no notice. Then all of a sudden the baby's head had come and I shouted, and of course they came running, and said, 'Why didn't you *say* you were having pains?' Then the sister was ever so cross, and they took the baby away and I didn't see her till six o'clock next morning. I didn't know if it was a boy or a girl, I didn't know if it was dead. Oh! I went through such agony of mind that night. Well – these things you just have to forget.[1]

It is not easy to forget though. Jean Robinson commented at a recent meeting that in letters received by the Patients' Association, depth of experience and length of memory made childbirth cases different from any other in her experience. Having a baby is not like having your appendix out. It is one of the most profound and important experiences in a woman's life.

Medical science, the domain of men, has therefore claimed childbirth as its own and yet refused to concern itself with those parts of the experience which are of vital importance to women. As one author of a book on psychiatric disorders in obstetrics puts it: 'There is no advantage for the patient in escaping a physical complication, merely to have her life made miserable by emotional problems.'[2] Obstetrics does not address itself to the quality of a woman's emotional experience of birth; emotional states belong to the psychiatrist. Nor does it concern itself with the quality of the newly delivered mother's relationship with her baby; that belongs to the paediatrician. The average layman may see all these things as inextricably connected but that does not make any difference to the way in which medical specialists operate within their own, jealously guarded territory. I remember attending a lecture given by a professor of obstetrics who was asked by a woman trying to form a postnatal support group how she should go about getting the backing of local obstetricians. She had, she explained, already won the support of psychiatrists in the area. The answer was immediate: 'Tell them you don't like the psychiatrists.' We must assume he knows his own kind.

The fact that these sober, professional men appear to behave rather like schoolboys on rival football teams has serious consequences for mothers. It means that our care throughout the whole birth experience from the first confirmation of pregnancy to the last postnatal visit six weeks after birth is divided amongst different groups of specialists, none of whom is specifically responsible for detecting and treating postnatal depression.

It is confusing to have to deal with a series of strange

'experts' and I shall be dealing more fully with the important issue of continuity of care in Chapter 7. It is enough to say here that during the course of my first pregnancy and labour, which were dealt with entirely by the hospital, my body was touched and handled by no fewer than fifteen different people, only three of whom asked my permission or bothered to explain who they were or what they were doing. This is by no means unusual. Hospitals assume control of our bodies from the point where we enter their doors. We become patients who have a particular role to play within an autonomous institution run according to its own authoritarian rules. We are told to put ourselves completely in the hands of the staff because they are 'the experts'. We are expected to obey regulations, without being told what the regulations are, and we are processed and delivered according to a set procedure which we may not need but over which we have no control.

Daddy knows best. This is the paternal assumption of scientific obstetrics practised in its territory of sickness, the hospital. Women accept the assumption and conform to the role because the territory is alien, the atmosphere strange; the uniforms, machinery, instruments, even the beds proclaim efficiency, sterility and impending emergency: 'It was dark, the hospital was dark and cold and most of the lights were off, I suppose so the patients could go to sleep. It really sent a shiver up my back, being so dark and sombre. We went down to this cold, clean room with lots of instruments, it felt so cut off from everything.' In such an atmosphere birth does not seem like a happy event.

Is it fair to blame male doctors for this alienation? There are, after all, a large number of women working as nurses and midwives in maternity units. There are indeed, but the point at issue is not their presence but the degree of responsibility they hold. The hospital is a rigid hierarchical system, the kind of system which men always seem to create. Like a Christmas tree it spreads its branches broadly at the bottom and the consultant shines like a star at the top.

The position which each group holds within the hierarchy is very important to them. Beneath the consultant are the senior registrars, senior house officers and house officers on the medical side, not to mention students if they are around. All these wear white coats. Beneath them on the lower branches come the nursing staff, many of whom are also midwives; they wear different coloured uniforms. There is sister and her staff nurses, state registered nurses, state enrolled nurses, student nurses, pupil nurses and nursing auxiliaries.

Within this hospital hierarchy, the greatest pressure is felt by those at the bottom. Nurses are given little initiative. Certain routines are observed quite divorced from their original purpose, i.e. to keep the patient clean and comfortable. Just as children infuriate mothers by creating work, washing, cleaning up, tidying, so patients create work for nurses.

Another nurse said: 'We can't let her have it [the baby] yet – we haven't taken the nailbrushes round the wards and Matron is on her way.'[3]

A few minutes later I felt sick and rang to ask for a bowl. She was busy, could I wait a bit? I was humiliatingly sick on the sheet which she insisted, crossly, on changing though I suggested apologetically that she could just sponge it. I was clearly being a nuisance.[4]

She was terribly cross every time the undersheet got wet (with leaking membranes). She said, 'The doctor's coming you know, any minute now.'

In their book on hospitals, *Communicating with the Patient*, P. Ley and M. S. Spelman write: 'It is argued that hospital staff see patients as beings with no rights, who should be grateful for any attention that they receive. Gerda Cohen suggests that these attitudes are hangovers from "Poor Law" regimes . . . In the eyes of the staffs of some hospitals, patients appear to be at the bottom of a rigid hierarchy.'[5] I think the examples I have given above amply illustrate this. In a situation where master kicks servant and servant kicks dog, the patient becomes the dog. In theory of course the dog can bite back, but given that women as a whole are easily intimidated and that even the most self-assured woman is at her most desperately vulnerable in labour and the week or so following, it is likely that the emotional reaction to these sorts of experiences will be felt by the baby and the husband. The institution is impervious because the institution has no feelings.

The midwives who work in maternity units have a very limited area of responsibility and little room for manoeuvre within it. They cannot protect the woman giving birth from procedures which distress her because those procedures are dictated by people farther up the tree. They see a constant stream of strange women passing through like a conveyor belt: shave, enema, bath, examine, wait, deliver, move on; shave, enema, bath, examine . . . The system iself prevents real human contact and at this level it is serviced by people who are overworked and underpaid.

The district midwife, on the other hand, is equally overworked and underpaid but has far more independence and initiative. She is not working within a rigid hierarchy in an institution removed from the community. She is a familiar and respected figure in the district dealing with mothers she knows in their own homes where each feels special and important.

This explains, in part, the callousness, indifference and sometimes downright punitive attitudes displayed too often by women as nurses and midwives to women as patients who are pregnant, in labour or newly delivered:

> This backache was getting worse and worse. They said the backache was because the baby was facing the wrong way, his head was pressing on my back. I said to the midwife, 'Would you please rub my back,' because basically that's all I wanted. She was at that time standing up against the wall waiting for things to happen and she said, 'Why?', and in my confused state I thought, 'Why is she asking why?, she must know why, because I hurt,' and I said, 'Please, please would you rub my back.' And her face set. She said, 'I haven't got the time.'

This kind of callousness is difficult to forgive, but it is easy to see how it can arise within the framework I have outlined. In his book *Human Aggression* Anthony Storr comments: 'Perhaps our most unpleasant characteristic as a species is our proclivity for bullying the helpless.'[6] In the same way that a tired, discouraged mother will strike out at a small child who is making emotional demands she cannot meet, so the harassed midwife hits out at the woman in labour. There is also the strong cultural undercurrent that women *should* suffer during labour, a hangover from the 'pregnancy as punishment' attitudes towards sex. As one antenatal teacher with years of experience explained to me:

> Midwives and nurses don't say, 'Oh, you are clever dear, you are doing beautifully,' they say, 'Come along Mrs So-and-So, pull yourself together, you've got hours to go. What are you going to be like when it *really* hurts?' It doesn't happen in Holland does it? In Holland midwives and doctors enjoy women having babies, they think it's great. They like birth, they think it's a nice and proper physiological event and it should happen in the home – and we don't. I blame our medical system. We must give midwives some status, give them credit for the skills they've got. Hospital midwives are just so shat upon, they've got to take it out on somebody. Well, who do you take it out on, if not that bloody silly woman who's screaming her head off and all she's doing is having a baby for Christ's sake!

In a large, impersonal, streamlined system there is not much room for compassion, tenderness or joy. The mystery which surrounds birth, the sense of the renewal of life is lacking in most labour wards because they exist to perform a technical function. As one doctor told me: 'Medicine is initially a technical operation which involves doing the bare technical necessities and when it comes to childbirth the technical operation is getting the baby out alive and keeping the mother alive and getting them home, and that's it.' Given such a strictly technical definition of birth, it is easy to see how the woman as a person becomes redefined as a functioning uterus with all the alienation involved in that. Doctors are technicians, that is their training, anything else is a pure accident of personality and disposition. No obstetrician was ever examined on his attitude to women! We may hope and expect that doctors will be sensitive to us but there is nothing in their training that guarantees it.

Sheila Kitzinger writes of the doctor-patient relationship: 'It need not be a blind leaning on the obstetrician's superior wisdom. It can mean the woman's intelligent participation, in which she works as part of a team, and in which the woman is playing not the role of a child but of an adult participating in a vital life process.'[7] Her positive and hopeful view is not reflected in the tone of the BMA publication, *You and Your Baby*: 'You are going to have to answer a lot of questions and be the subject of a lot of examinations. Never worry year head about any of these.'[8] (It seems our heads aren't pretty and little any more.)

One woman informed her obstetrician that she was having Braxton Hicks contractions (painless contractions felt at the end of pregnancy). 'What do *you* know about Braxton Hicks contractions?' he said, alarmed. 'I'm having them,' she replied. Her intelligent participation was unwelcome. Actually the woman who tries to establish herself as a participating adult risks more than a rebuff, she risks being labelled 'masculine' and that is a fate worse than death, for we are informed by a consultant obstetrician: 'From *a purely biological aspect* the masculine type of female and the effeminate type of male are not good vehicles for the reproduction and the procreation of the human race.'[9] (My italics.) A comment which could be regarded as fascist it is so dangerously prejudiced. Biology defines male and female, culture defines masculine and feminine. If her ovaries and womb are in good working order a woman is quite capable of bearing a normal, healthy baby whether she is a tough business executive, a butch lesbian, a hearty horsewoman, an aggressive feminist or any other 'masculine type of female'.

The fact that doctors can make such silly remarks simply reflects the extent to which their general education has been neglected. The average liberal arts student at university probably knows far more about sociology, psychology and sex than the medical student who will later make decisions involving a knowledge of all three. There are some who believe that the only students worthy of public support are students of medicine and engineering. It is important to remember, however, that the study of the humanities is the study of the nature of man in his languages, social organization, economic organization, history, anthropology, early development and learning and expression of subjective experience through art and literature. Medicine studies none of these; like engineering it studies a functioning machine and increasingly the human body is talked of as a machine (heart-pump, brain-computer) when in fact it is the machine which copies the body not the body which is a machine.

There was a time when medicine was placed firmly amongst the humanities, but that is no longer so. It is now a science and increasingly involved with technology. What medical students need is more imaginative experience of other people's lives and values, for handling the human body never was like mending a car and never will be.

The average medical student is male, probably from a medical (upper middle-class) family and public school (single sex) educated. At university medics are usually segregated from students in other disciplines in separate buildings. The course is very rigorous so there is little time for general reading and discussion. It is no coincidence that the stereotype medical student behaves like a larky schoolboy; engineering students who work on equally heavy fact-learning specialist courses tend to behave in the same way. Given this kind of background and training, it is not surprising if a doctor's ideas about human behaviour in general and female psychology in particular are limited.

There are remarkable exceptions and a growing number of them, but on the whole obstetricians still treat women as frightened children and emotional dependence is encouraged in the name of trust. This might not be so bad if they were dependable, but like most men they are afraid of emotion. The following story illustrates this very well:

There was a foreign girl, a Persian girl, who was being examined and she cried, I heard her from the other cubicle. I think they were taking a smear with this steel thing. He kept saying, '*Oh, don't cry so much, you'll worry the*

other patients.' She was a foreign girl and obviously it
was the first time in her life that any other man but her
husband had entered her. She was heart-broken. I could hear
the most stifling sobs and I thought, 'You are a bit of a
brute you know. If you had any imagination you would
just treat it with so much more care, because she's a human
being.'

The girl's cries were obviously worrying the doctor far more
than the other patients and yet he was unable to cope
with the emotional situation. His scientific training provided
him with no resources, so he was compelled to rely on an
authoritarian pose.

The vagina is a sexual organ. Any internal examination
is a sexual act. This is true of the doctor doing it and the
woman receiving it. In one story I was told, a woman was
examined by the doctor who said, 'I'm afraid you're very
bruised Mrs O'Flynn'; 'What do you expect!' said she. 'What
do you expect! You used two fingers, O'Flynn only uses one.'
Perhaps it would be better if we could be as forthright about
the situation. As it is, most women dread the public display
of their private parts and all the 'poking and prodding' they
are subjected to.

One GP explained to me that obstetricians are very shy
men. If this is true, it may explain why they so often appear
aloof, clinical and uncommunicative. Lack of communication is one of the things which worry women most when they
are having a baby. Bad communication is not exclusive to
maternity wards but it is felt more. In her research for *Human
Relations and Hospital Care*, Ann Cartwright discovered that
maternity patients more often than others wanted to know all
about their condition, including details. One report from her
book illustrates what so often happens: 'Well I was worried
whether having this stuff in my water would affect the baby,
but the sister just said, "You're worrying yourself unduly. You
should leave these things to us." But I don't think she thought
I could understand. I think she thought I wasn't educated
enough.'[10] Daddy knows best again.

One mother wrote to me describing a similar experience:

'I was examined and left in a side ward with another woman. My husband was sent home. I asked if it was a breech presentation and was told "not to worry", and then to be quiet as I would wake other patients by talking!' She was a woman who, after two miscarriages and a difficult pregnancy with a query breech presentation (baby coming bottom first) went into labour a month early. She was later heavily drugged: 'They told me I wasn't progressing and gave me a pethidine injection. I was amazed. I was coping well and I wanted to move around, but no, I had to lie down. Anyway three injections later the baby was born by forceps delivery.' As a result of the drugs her baby was dopey and would not feed: 'Then on the eighth day the baby actually woke up and went to the breast. I cried. On the tenth day I went home, still crying. For the next six months I cried. The tiredness got worse, the crying got worse. It was awful.'

Being told not to worry and being subjected to procedures without proper explanation is no help at all. It creates anxiety and alienation. Nor is this something which happens only in the supercharged emergency atmosphere of the labour ward:

> I had pains, frequent abdominal pains and I assumed I was set for a miscarriage all the way through . . . but what annoyed me was that my doctor, and he's a very good doctor actually, he would never tell me anything about these pains, he would never sort of pay much attention to them and I felt that he thought I was, you know, that they weren't really there and so that annoyed me really and I still to this day don't know what the wretched pains were or whether I did in fact threaten miscarriage or not.

On the other hand, good communication can have very beneficial results: 'I felt very calm before the birth, thanks to an excellent gynaecologist who explained everything that was happening; he also included my husband in discussions if he happened to be there, and so I felt I had a great deal of support.'

So why is communication so bad in hospitals? Who is

responsible for explaining to women what is happening? Is *anyone* actually responsible? How do the different branches of the tree communicate with each other? In an authoritarian structure where orders are passed down the line, it is not to be expected that a nurse would speculate on something as technical as a breech presentation even if the doctor is not there. There is also the deliberate medical mystique which surrounds the process; doctors do not want us to know too much about it. Yet again, Daddy knows best. But, we might ask, does he really know what is going on?

A group of consultant obstetricians were shown a film (made by Helen Brew with a commentary by R. D. Laing) about the damaging effects of current obstetric procedures on both the emotional state of the mother and the relationship she forms with her baby. Afterwards one consultant was heard to comment that he didn't really understand it, all that his mothers seemed to worry about was getting nannies. Few National Health Service patients have such worries!

Another consultant obstetrician has written:

> Such a comparatively simple remark like, 'My dear, I suppose there is nothing that can be done about it at this stage, but they did leave Mary Jane alone for hours' is the type of comment that it is impossible to disprove and will require massive reassurance to correct. If it is not corrected, even just a niggling thought two or three times a day that perhaps one might be left alone for hours in labour is detrimental to the trust and confidence a woman should have at this time. Probably more is done by wicked women with their malicious lying tongues to harm the confidence and happiness of pregnant women than by any other single factor.[11]

Strong stuff that, and yet Ann Cartwright comments on her survey:

> Three fifths of the maternity patients were left alone at some stage during their labour, and this proportion was 69 per cent among mothers having their first baby. Although

a few mothers prefer to be on their own, others were worried and upset by their isolation, and as a group those who were left alone were more critical of the nurses than were those who had someone with them all the time.[12]

Despite political promises that less pressure on the maternity services (and schools come to that) would lead to improved conditions, in fact the opposite has happened. The sharp decline in the birth rate has led to economic cut-backs which have often meant staff shortages, closure of small local maternity hospitals, and for some women a fifty-mile journey to get to the nearest large hospital. Women who do not have their husbands with them complain of being left alone in labour as much today as they did in the past.[13]

One of the side-effects of the medical scientific take-over of the birth process is that it becomes very difficult to alter procedures once they are instituted. Women are not given a choice as to whether they are shaved, bathed, have enemas or have episiotomies. Women are not even allowed to decide whether they want to stand up, sit down, walk or lie during labour. All are expected to lie flat. They are certainly not allowed to have anyone they want with them. Husbands may now be allowed, if not always actually welcomed, but it would be a very unusual hospital which allowed an unmarried father or a friend, relative or neighbour to be present.

As a consequence one group of men have to go away and conduct a great deal of research to prove that the procedures instituted by another group of men are unhelpful and not what women want. One example of this is the research which has been done into the position of the body during labour.

In all primitive societies and in our own up to the advent of the man-midwives in the early nineteenth century, women always gave birth standing, squatting or kneeling. It appears that, left to their own devices, women were well able to appreciate the benefits of the law of gravity. Man-midwives entered the birth scene chiefly as surgeons at difficult deliveries. Their tool was the forceps, for years kept a closely guarded secret. They persuaded women to lie flat on their backs when they gave birth since this was easier for them, the man-midwives. So it began, and so it continues. One doctor who has done much research into the subject is Dr Caldeyro-Barcia, president of the International Federation of Gynae-cologists and Obstetricians, and he is quoted as saying, 'Except for being hung by the feet, the supine position is the worst conceivable position for labour and delivery.'

Needless to say, one finding of all this research is that women *prefer* standing, sitting, kneeling or walking during labour rather than lying prone hour after hour. But then who would dream of giving women the choice, except during a research project of course! One woman I talked to sorted it out for herself: 'When I was having him I was further on than they realized. I just kept going to the toilet and sitting on it and I found that was really helpful.'

This is one example of the way in which men conduct research to convince other men to change practices which female common sense and experience could have told them were harmful in the first place. Another example is the research done by Marshall H. Klaus and John H. Kennell, two American paediatricians at Case Western Reserve University, Cleveland, Ohio, into mother-baby bonding during the first hour after birth. They have discovered that it is very important to the future relationship of mother and baby that the newborn should be given to her mother as soon as possible and for as long as possible after birth. But midwives never used to separate mother and baby. It was clean, safe science and men in their hospitals who thought that one up and, as I know from personal experience, they will not change their minds however often they are asked by a mother. It takes pages of scientific proof to alter an inhuman procedure undertaken in the name of science.

After all that research it is a relief to turn to yet another man, Dr Frederick Leboyer, who presents his plea for birth without violence in a more poetic vein:

After all this, I can say only one thing: 'Try.'
Everything that has been said here is simple. So simple that one feels embarrassed at having dwelt upon it at such length. Perhaps we have lost our taste for simplicity. Here,

we need so little. None of these expensive gadgets for monitoring, none of the technologist's modish products.

Only a little patience and humility. A little silence. Unobtrusive but real attention. Awareness of the newcomer as a person. Unself-consciousness.

And love.[14]

5. Science and Technology

Prevention can be worse than cure.

In mental hospitals at the turn of the century patients who were thought to be suicide risks were kept locked up, naked, in padded cells with no objects of any kind with which to damage themselves. They were escorted closely whenever they left their cells. Incredibly, despite all this, some of them still managed to kill themselves.

Humane psychiatrists noted that by stripping these patients of all human dignity 'just in case' they killed themselves, they were not only being unhelpful, they were actually making the condition worse. The practice was stopped. A degree of risk was accepted.

To live is to risk. Without risk we are all living in that padded cell. Prevention has a break-even point. Up to that point it is helpful, beyond that point it can be harmful. Obstetrics has now passed its break-even point.

There is a curious psychology to prevention. Often, by being over-anxious about a particular risk we can actually make the accident more likely. This is marvellously illustrated in a children's book, *Mary-Mary*:

> One day Mary-Mary started coming downstairs backwards, pulling a box of bricks behind her.
>
> Miriam, Martyn, Mervyn and Meg were all standing together in the hall, and when they heard Mary-Mary coming *bumpety-bump* down the stairs backwards they all started shouting at her at once:
>
> 'Don't come down backwards, Mary-Mary. You'll fall down!'
>
> Mary-Mary fell down. And all the bricks came after her.
> 'There!' said Miriam. 'We said you'd fall down.'
> 'There!' said Martyn. 'We knew you would.'
> 'There!' said Mervyn. 'Just as we said.'
> 'There!' said Meg. 'What did we tell you?'

'You told me to fall down,' said Mary-Mary, 'and I think it was very silly of you.'[1]

The very atmosphere of emergency in a high technology hospital can create the kind of conditions it is there to prevent, as this woman's experience shows: 'I had rather high blood pressure every time I went to the hospital clinic (it was OK when my own doctor checked it!) and they kept threatening me with bed rest in hospital. That did upset me and I broke down in tears a few times at the clinic. I wasn't at all keen on going into hospital to have the baby and resting there wouldn't have helped.' It is difficult to feel relaxed in an atmosphere which is felt to be threatening.

The use of technology only became an important issue in the birth field as late as the 1970s. Before that induction meant enema, hot bath, castor oil or artificially rupturing the membranes (bag of water surrounding the foetus) and waiting. Before that monitoring meant a midwife or doctor listening to the foetal heartbeat through a special trumpet-like foetal stethoscope. During the 1970s induction came to mean the use of an oxytocin drug passed through a drip into a vein of the arm and monitoring came to mean being wired up to two machines, one monitoring the strength of contractions through a metal disc strapped round the abdomen and the other monitoring the foetal heartbeat by means of wires passed up the vagina and attached to the skull of the foetus.

The difference between these methods in terms of mobility, self-control and simple, old-fashioned human dignity is considerable.

If these new techniques were used only in those cases where there were genuine obstetric complications they might justly have been heralded as a genuine medical advance. But they were not. Doctors spread their nets wider and wider as their enthusiasm for their new techniques increased.

In 1971 when I had my first baby I met no one who had been monitored by machine. In 1974 when I had my second baby I found that every labour in that same hospital was being so monitored. The same thing was happening with induction. Increasingly the new technique was being used for social reasons, so that babies could be born during day-light hours. Even when induction itself was not necessary, doctors were using the oxytocin drip to 'speed up' labours which had started naturally but seemed to be going rather slowly.

In October 1974 the *Sunday Times* ran two feature articles by their medical correspondent called 'The Childbirth Revolution,' which were followed in January 1975 by a BBC *Horizon* documentary on induction called 'A Time to be Born' and in February of that year by a series of articles in the *Sun* newspaper called 'Assembly Line Babies'. The public debate had started. It has not yet finished.

Why did obstetrics decide to interfere with normal, healthy births? They had never, historically, been much interested in normal birth up to that point, they had delegated it to the midwives. The arguments they use are that this is a logical extension of preventative medicine. These procedures are carried out 'just in case' something goes wrong. Just in case labour takes too long, it will be speeded up; just in case the foetus becomes distressed it will be monitored; just in case the perineum tears it will be cut. All is done in an attempt to produce an ideal, British Standard labour which doesn't exist in nature.

This 'active management of labour' has also been called 'aggressive obstetrics' because it attacks first without waiting to see if there is any real need. There is danger to the baby in all this; some induced babies have been born premature; contractions produced by the oxytocin drip may be too strong, thus creating foetal distress requiring an emergency Caesarean operation; electrodes attached to the scalp of the foetus may create an abscess. And so, in order to try and minimize the risks of one procedure, other procedures are introduced.

Technology breeds technology. The contractions produced by an oxytocin drip may be too strong and therefore must be monitored; there may be foetal distress as a result so the foetal heartbeat must be monitored. The contractions may be too strong for the mother to tolerate so she should be given epidural analgesia, which may mean that she will be unable to push the baby out later because she does not feel the contractions and therefore forceps will be needed.

Thus a perfectly healthy woman who has gone into labour spontaneously may find herself lying immobilized, with a drip in her arm, a tube in her spine, a strap round her middle and wires up her vagina. How does that make her feel?

They tried to inject me against my will, conned me into having an oxytocin drip (I read my notes later and was furious!) by telling me rudely that it was glucose. I so much wanted to have my baby naturally . . . I would never, never go into hospital again.

They strapped me round the middle with rather horrible rubber tubes and a sort of plate in the middle of my stomach. Then my contractions started coming fairly thick and fast and it wasn't long before I said, 'Would you take this thing off me please.' And this night nurse said, 'We can't.' I thought, 'I've *got* to get out of this thing,' because I was really getting claustrophobic. With the tension of the contractions I was really beginning to feel hysterical.

Both these reactions show that the procedures used had a strong emotional effect and it is the emotional reaction to aggressive obstetrics which concerns me in this book. As one psychiatrist commented to me: 'Somebody's got to ask the question, at what point should it stop? What effect does it have on a woman to have wires inside the vagina while she's having a baby when in fact there shouldn't be wires there. How do we balance the equation between a baby's heart stopping and a mother's mind freaking?' This is a very important question and since the obstetricians responsible for dealing with the first half of that equation are apparently not on speaking terms with the psychiatrists dealing with the second half, it must be the community who decides at what point it should stop. Hospitals are not insensitive to public opinion.

Dana Breen, in her research into the factors which lead to a good adjustment to motherhood, studied fifty-one women having first babies. Using Pitt's depression questionnaire as one of her research tools, she found that seventeen women were depressed (ill-adjusted) and thirty-four were not (well-adjusted) and comments that the women who coped well with having a baby were those who could feel they were active and creative while doing so: 'Of foremost importance is the woman's feeling that her body is able to be productive, that it is able to "give" birth to her baby.'[2] This feeling of initiation and activity was in strong contrast to the sense of passivity of the poorly adjusted group.

Having your labour actively managed is, by definition, a passive experience. The management, control and creativity of the act of birth are removed from the hands of the mother and taken into the hands of the doctor. If, as a result, a woman's confidence in herself as a woman and a mother is shattered; if she feels she has failed and is inadequate, then depression is just around the corner, putting both mother and baby at risk. Dana Breen gives an example of this:

> With her first child she was induced on the day the baby was due for no urgent obstetrical reason and delivered three days later with a vacuum extraction. 'As I was coming down, I said to the doctor: "Well, I couldn't even manage that on my own . . ." ' Although she had planned to breast-feed, when the time came she didn't feel able to ask to breastfeed; she felt she had failed at giving birth, how could she possibly manage to feed the baby from her own body? She became depressed and did not want another baby for some years. The birth of her second child, on the contrary, was straightforward. She had no problem breast-feeding this second baby . . . Even one year after the birth of her second child she still polarizes her feelings towards the two children, the one who makes her feel so inadequate and the one who makes her feel such a good mother.[3]

Why did this woman come to feel inadequate? Was the induction 'for no urgent obstetrical reason' worth the risk in terms of its emotional repercussions for both mother and child? Who tried to balance that equation?

One person who does try is Dr Desmond Bardon, who has written: 'The other serious and tardily acknowledged dangers arising from accelerated labour are interference with the mutual attachment of mother and child and damage to the mother's confidence in herself as a mother and as a woman.'[4] This comes from a letter written to the *British Medical Journal* in response to an article printed there. The *BMJ* did not choose to publish it.

There has been no research into a possible relationship between the experience of childbirth and postnatal depression. There is plenty of evidence that many current obstetric procedures can and do contribute to depression in individual cases but this is not statistical proof.

Brice Pitt in his study in 1968 found that there was no connection between depression and pregnancy complications or between depression and a complicated delivery. His findings are supported by Katharina Dalton's research in 1971. She mentions that the depressives tend to have considered their labours to be more difficult, but the difference was not statistically significant. Both studies took place before the widespread use of birth technology.

One study which could have proved something, was that commissioned by the Department of Health and Social Security and undertaken by Ann Cartwright, into mothers' experiences of induction. This study makes an analysis of over 2000 random births in 24 areas of England and Wales. Unfortunately, however, no distinction is made between mothers who were induced by means of the oxytocin drip and mothers induced by other methods (such as artificial rupturing of the membranes). Nor is any information given about the numbers of women in the non-induced group who had accelerated labours. Comparison is therefore impossible, since a labour started spontaneously and then controlled by a drip is likely to be experienced in a similar way to a labour induced and controlled by a drip. What it is important to discover is the difference in experience between a normal labour in which there is no interference and an actively managed labour with modern obstetric technology.

There are three interesting facts which her study does reveal, however. One is that 78 per cent of those having an induction would prefer not to have another, the main reason being that they would prefer 'the baby to come naturally'. Women, it would seem, do not want birth to become a medically-managed event.

Another interesting fact was that in 37 hospitals at which 20 or more of the study births occurred, the proportion of inductions ranged from 0 per cent to 57 per cent. This shows that there are very considerable differences between hospitals in the practices they use. The third point of interest and a very important one was that 71 per cent of all mothers having vaginal deliveries also had episiotomies.[5]

An episiotomy is a cut in the perineum which is made at the time of delivery. Doctors say that this cut is made in cases where there is a risk that there will be a tear. A cut is cleaner and easier to stitch than a jagged tear. It has increasingly been claimed, however, that episiotomies are performed as a matter of routine, 'just in case' there is a tear. A figure of 71 per cent in such a large study supports that claim.

Does it matter? To the doctor apparently not, since it is done so frequently. To the woman, her husband and her baby it can matter a great deal. The pain of stitches following birth are considered by some women as the worst part of the whole experience: 'The worst part of the birth was the stitches, I found them agony.' Being constantly in pain whether standing, sitting or lying at a time when we already have more than enough to cope with has obvious repercussions:

Because I was in agony all the time I was not interested in the baby because I blamed him for the pain I was in.[6]

This experience ruined our first three months. My husband was very understanding but was beginning to think I was making excuses for not having intercourse, and this was also worrying me.[7]

Episiotomy has been called 'the unkindest cut' because

the perineum is such an incredibly sensitive sexual area which can take a long time to heal, even when it has been stitched properly. Delay in resuming sex because of the pain is common. In one survey, delay varied from two months to two years. This is a situation which is hardly designed to promote family happiness at a time of stress. On occasion things can go so badly wrong that they precipitate a breakdown:

> A student doctor was standing by to stitch me up afterwards. When he found he was unable to do the job a doctor was called and took an hour and a half to stitch. He was concerned that I may not have been stitched properly. When I returned to the hospital for the six week check-up, the doctor, a different one, told me that I had been stitched tightly and may have trouble with sexual intercourse. We did have trouble, it was impossible. When eventually I went back into hospital for the plastic surgery operation my son was seven months old. I had been breast-feeding him but had to stop. Taking all this into account I was obviously upset, which eventually culminated in a nervous breakdown.[8]

We must hope that this woman's episiotomy was not done simply as a matter of routine.

Having avoided an episiotomy with my first baby because the student was not quick enough with his scissors and been given one with my second baby because the doctor was, I can only say that there was no comparison between the two experiences. With my first baby I had a very slight tear in the vagina which was stitched but caused no pain or discomfort afterwards. My sex life was not affected at all. With the episiotomy, which was well stitched, there was acute pain and discomfort for months. I felt I had been assaulted. It took a long time for my sex life to return to normal. It took a long time for me to start liking my body again.

Episiotomy should *never* be performed as a matter of routine, it is simply not necessary. In Holland, where 50 per cent of births still take place at home, the proportion of episiotomies performed is 6 per cent. Are we to believe that Dutch women are anatomically different from British women, or is it simply that their attendants have more patience, and more faith in normal birth?

Impatience is the enemy of the natural birth process. Impatience leads to active management of labour and continual interference. It seems that doctors cannot watch and wait, help and support, be still. Men must act, control, perform; this is nothing new:

> As Dr Matthews Duncan said at the end of his course in Obstetrics, 'I have been lecturing to you for many weeks on the science and art of obstetrics. I wonder if any of you realize what is the *hardest* thing to do in midwifery? It is to do nothing. Further, I wonder if you realize what is the *most important* thing to do in midwifery? It is to do nothing.'

This quotation comes from a lecture given in 1922 by the New Zealand psychiatrist Frederick Truby King, the once influential and now totally discredited child-care expert. He adds his own comment: 'If the maternal death-rate is to be lowered, medical men must realize that forceps should not be clamped on because the hands of the clock approach eleven p.m.'[9] That has a familiar ring to it. The tools may have changed but the desire to abuse them has not. Ever since the man-midwife entered the birth scene he has sought to improve on nature. In cases of abnormal birth this has been of great value. Looking back on the history of obstetric science, we have much to be grateful for, but science should be the servant of nature, not her master; the birth attendant should attend not the machine but the mother:

> After a while the sister midwife came along and turned the machine round because she said it was distracting (which it was). Also, she had a word with the nurses and told them they should be caring for me, and observing me, not constantly watching the machine – that was not midwifery.[10]

This mother had a good birth.

In the debate which has raged round the issues involved in the active management of labour the doctors, not surprisingly, compare the situation to that of other operations. We do not, they point out, expect continuity of care when we have our tonsils out. We do not expect to have our appendix removed by a junior doctor (a comparison with midwives). Why apply different rules to birth? Why indeed, if birth is a medical condition comparable to dangerously enlarged tonsils or a diseased appendix.

But it is not. Birth is a natural life event. As such it is directly comparable with sex. Some people have sexual problems which require medical help, be it physical or psychiatric. The majority of us manage without and are not considered to be in danger.

This was not always the case. Sexual activity was, during Victorian times, regarded as a highly dangerous thing to be actively discouraged. Doctors became quite hysterical about the dangers of masturbation which, they claimed, could lead to blindness, insanity and moral deterioration. Alex Comfort in his book *The Anxiety Makers* quotes one of the medical arguments used for the surgical removal of the female clitoris in the interests of health:

> But girls have been neglected . . . I do feel an irresistible impulse to cry out against the shameful neglect of the clitoris and its hood, because of the vast amount of sickness and suffering which could have been saved the gentler sex, if this important subject received proper attention and appreciation at the hands of the profession. Circumcision for the girl or woman at any age is as necessary as for the boy or man.[11]

Female castration advocated as preventative medicine – and is routine episiotomy so very different?

Sexual activity was reclaimed from the area of sickness partly by changing social attitudes following the First World

War; partly by the work of Freud and his disciples and finally by the publication of the Kinsey Report as late as 1950 which revealed that masturbation is the most universal of sexual activities. Sex has returned to the community; will birth do the same?

The legacy of guilt and fear associated with masturbation is with us still. The legacy of reliance on obstetric technology has yet to be assessed. What is most worrying is that doctors and midwives alike, by distrusting the natural birth process and relying heavily on sophisticated equipment, are losing their traditional skills, their ability to judge what is happening by eyes, hand and intuition. Are machines as reliable?

> ، . . the machine was not behaving too well, and my husband, an electronics engineer, was helping to adjust it.[12]

> . . . When I was given an internal examination, the nurse removed the electrode and the machine stopped, then the nurse panicked and went screaming to the sister and doctor that the heartbeat had stopped.[13]

The traditional skills of midwifery born of long experience and shrewd judgement are too precious to be lost. They are skills which will be needed if women are to retain some control over how, when and where they have their babies. Nor is the tossing around of statistics much use in the argument; as John Davis, a paediatrician, has said: 'We are not dealing with matters that are susceptible to statistical analysis.'[14]

Indeed we are not. Someone has got to ask the question, at what point should it stop? An American doctor, in an article revealingly called 'The medical case against natural childbirth', defends the use of general anaesthetic in the second stage of labour: 'The only "natural phenomenon" that anaesthesia prevents is the expulsive stage of labour, a stage that is best controlled by the doctor, not the patient.' Since the expulsive stage of labour is birth itself it is of course a very important 'natural phenomenon'. He further comments on the use of forceps: 'The low forceps is so vital a part of good obstetrics that deliveries in which it is used are now classified statistically as "normal" rather than "operative".[15]

If forceps can be classified as normal, how about Caesarean births? Suzanne Arms writes in *Immaculate Deception*:

> According to a nurse on the obstetrical team of a large teaching hospital in New York City, the rate of C-sections for one month in 1974 was an unbelievable 50 per cent.
>
> Could we be heading towards an era of the *routine* Caesarean birth? Why not? If the medical community establishes that surgical removal of the foetus is safer than other methods of birth, doctors may come to regard the Caesarean as the newest and best device available to 'bring those U.S. mortality statistics down'.[16]

And where America leads, is Britain far behind? So far we have been. We did not outlaw midwives as America did; we do not use general anaesthetics for delivery; we do not see forceps deliveries as normal; we do not strap women down to the delivery table during birth. But increasingly we do use the same technology, the same philosophy of active management, the same insistence that birth is an illness. So why not follow the process still further? Who knows but that with the astounding advances of medical science we may be able to eliminate risk altogether and dispense with dangerous, messy old nature:

> 'For of course,' said Mr Foster, 'in the vast majority of cases, fertility is merely a nuisance. One fertile ovary in twelve hundred – that would really be quite sufficient for our purposes. But we want to have a good choice. And of course one must always leave an enormous margin of safety. So we allow as many as thirty per cent of the female embryos to develop normally. The others get a dose of male sex-hormone every twenty-four metres for the rest of the course. Result: they're decanted as freemartins – structurally quite normal, but sterile. Guaranteed sterile. Which brings us at last,' continued Mr Foster, 'out of the realm of mere slavish imitation of nature into the much more interesting world of human invention.'

He rubbed his hands. For, of course, they didn't content themselves with merely hatching out embryos; any cow could do that.[17]

The hatcheries of Aldous Huxley's *Brave New World* are still in the future but they are a logical extension of the scientific control of birth as a technical process divorced from humanity.

If we are told by doctors that a refusal to have our labour interfered with is putting our happiness before the health of our baby, when that interference is a matter of 'just in case' routine, let it be quite clear, he is using one of the oldest forms of moral blackmail in the world.

It is the mother's responsibility to balance the risks to her baby's health against the risks to her own feelings and future relationship with her baby. It is unlikely that anyone in attendance will consider that equation to be important. The risks to the baby are minimal in women with normal healthy pregnancies; the psychological risks have yet to be assessed.

The decisions that women make will be different, for we have different sets of values and expectations. Some women find modern hospital birth very comforting: 'I found it exceedingly reassuring to be sort of cradled in the arms of the National Health Service and everything was being taken care of so beautifully.' Some women make a fuss and are subjected to considerable pressure and abuse. Some take avoiding action rather than suffer a confrontation: 'I stayed at home and took castor oil on the day I was due to go into hospital for an induction. I didn't want them doing the same things to me that I'd seen happen to other women.'[18] Some avoid induction by giving their hospitals the wrong dates; some stay at home as long as possible during the first stage of labour to avoid everything. Most have no idea what procedures are used in maternity units and do not know they have the right to refuse them.

A woman in labour is totally vulnerable. She is incapable of fight or flight; she is entirely at the mercy of her environment, which may be why most spontaneous deliveries occur in the hours of darkness, when the human animal is in least danger of attack. If her expectations of birth are not realized, she will feel a sense of loss; if her expectations of birth are not realized owing to meddlesome interference or callousness she will also feel cheated; a double loss. Loss is another basis of depression. It will be a fragment added to that stained glass window which need not have been there.

6. Birth and After Birth

When I was expecting my first baby I felt privileged to live in a country where excellent medical care and a free hospital bed were available to all women. When I was expecting my second baby I felt threatened, defensive and unhappy about that same medical system.

I acknowledge that compared to the pain and humiliation that many women suffer, my own experiences have been trivial. To me they mattered very much and I make no apology for that. I had prepared myself to cope with the viciousness of nature but was vulnerable to the callousness of Man.

Nature was kind to me. Both my pregnancies were boringly normal; I didn't even suffer from nausea, heartburn, varicose veins or any of the other 'minor ailments' which can make pregnancy an ordeal. My blood pressure was stable, my weight gain reasonable. My births were the same: both babies presented themselves the right way and both labours started spontaneously. I am one of the fortunate who gestate faster than the allotted forty weeks. Imogen was born two days before dates and Pippa a week; neither was premature. I never had to face induction.

When I first became pregnant I knew nothing about pregnancy or birth. I bought books. I attended antenatal classes at the hospital and at the National Childbirth Trust. I was fascinated by the whole process. I discovered that the hospital classes gave no information at all about the sensations and emotions of birth. The staff who gave the lectures seemed ill at ease in their role as teachers. Like children in a biology lesson we looked at medical diagrams, while our babies kicked inside us.

The NCT classes were very different. There was more time and fewer women. The teacher loved teaching and was excited by birth. We learned about the variety of sensations and emotions we might feel. We learned possible ways of coping with them. We discussed things together. I was never totally convinced that it would work for me but I enjoyed the classes and found the information invaluable. I felt confident and well prepared for labour.

The NCT has been attacked by conservative doctors and radical feminists alike. The doctors see it as radical and the feminists see it as conservative. Some doctors believe even the mildest female protest is feminist inspired but in fact the women's liberation movement in Britain has never been much interested in childbirth and is only now beginning to take the issues involved seriously. Knowledge is power. It is easier for a doctor to say induction is 'best for baby' than to defend a clinical decision. The work of the NCT is important in that it gives women the knowledge which enables them to feel in control of their bodies. Those doctors and midwives who see women as real people are not threatened by this.

My first labour was twenty-four hours or five hours, depending on where you start timing it. Like many first labours it started and stopped a great deal. It was on for two hours, off for five hours, on six hours, off six hours and then established for five hours to delivery. I didn't want to arrive at the hospital only to be sent home again, so I waited for my body to decide it really did intend to deliver the baby. I did some dusting, telephoned friends, read the paper. I was very happy. I didn't find the contractions painful, I expected them to get worse. I packed sandwiches and flasks of coffee for my husband, Richard. We arrived at the hospital at 8.15 p.m. and at 8.30, half-way through my routine enema, I started pushing the baby out. Imogen was born at 8.45, delivered by a midwife and a medical student. I felt ecstatic. We were all smiling. Richard looked as though he had been awarded a Nobel prize. We had the daughter we both desperately wanted. I was bright, alert and happy, just waiting to hold my baby . . .

And then the doctor arrived.

I had never seen him before. He was thin and had ginger hair. He looked starchy and peeved. 'You were in a hurry,' he said, trying to be jocular. We all felt uneasy. He checked the baby and declared her healthy and well.

'Can I hold her?' I asked. No reply.

'Can she hold the baby?' Richard asked. 'Later,' he said. I waited.

'Can I feed her?' I tried. He laughed.

'*She's* not hungry,' he sneered.

My joy evaporated and vanished. I knew he was wrong. I knew the suckling instinct is strongest in the newborn and I had colostrum to give her. I also knew intuitively there was no way that that man would *allow* me to hold and love my baby and in that environment his authority was absolute. I betrayed myself and my child in that I didn't fight; I hadn't thought I should need to. He destroyed for me what might have been a perfect birth and with it the trust I'd had in the goodwill of doctors.

> In summary, we hypothesize that there is a sensitive period in the human mother which is the optimal time for an affectional bond to develop between the mother and her infant. The suggestion that mother-infant contact and interaction in the early minutes and hours after delivery influence subsequent mothering behaviour is supported by the results in six of these eight controlled studies of mothers of premature infants and parents of full-term infants.[1]

This rather ponderous and dry statement comes from a paper by Klaus and Kennell called 'Evidence for a sensitive period in the human mother'. It is the kind of statement of which doctors take notice. Indeed, like tablets from the mountain the results of their research have been received as a great revelation. The simple request of a newly delivered mother to hold and feed her baby is easily dismissed. A controlled study with supporting statistics is 'scientific'. Unfortunately for me, Klaus and Kennell had not completed their studies in December 1971 when Imogen was born.

Finally, two hours after my baby was born, I saw her and held her for the brief five minutes it took to wheel me to the postnatal wards when she was again removed to the nursery and I was left to sleep.

It was the week before Christmas and everything was re-laxed and cheerful in the postnatal wards. I didn't find being in hospital much of a rest for the daily routine was too complicated, and advice contradictory. I was discharged on Christmas Eve and pleased to be home.

I wanted to have my second baby at home. I wanted to include Imogen in the birth as she was included in the pregnancy. I wanted to feel confident that I could hold my baby and have her with me from the moment she was born. Richard was unhappy about the idea of home birth and I didn't press the issue. I didn't know then that aggressive obstetrics had arrived in Britain.

I was booked in for a hospital confinement but my GP shared my antenatal care. I liked that very much. I liked sitting in the waiting-room with young girls and old men, toddlers and teenagers. I shared their coughs and swollen glands and aching feet; they shared my baby. I liked being in the doctor's surgery with its absolute privacy. I liked the knowledge that his care for the baby inside would continue when she was outside.

I went to the hospital once or twice. All the doctors had changed but they were pleasant enough. It was smooth and uneventful until the seventh month. Then I noticed that friends who had had apparently normal labours were reporting their experiences of 'machines'. I asked my GP what was going on. He said the hospital was engaged in a research programme using foetal monitoring machines on all women in labour. He told me I had every right to object and in case the hospital was difficult he wrote me a letter.

I suspect his letter saved me from a great deal of pressure. The obstetrician at the hospital was very patient. He explained how fortunate I was to have this technology available to me. He explained that the hospital liked live babies. He did not explain why the hospital was not informing women about their programme. I didn't even attempt to explain why I objected. He would not have understood that I was fighting to protect my baby and give her a happy birth.

With my first baby I had taken it for granted that the ideal situation which everyone hoped for was a normal, spontaneous, undrugged labour. I had been lucky, I had managed to have that and had found it an intense and joyful experience. With my second baby I could not take it for granted that my view of birth was shared. My desire to give birth to my second baby as I had my first was suddenly peculiar and deviant. I became hostile, defensive and increasingly anxious about having this baby in hospital. I longed to crawl into a dark, warm cupboard and give birth in a basket like a cat.

I arrived late at the hospital with my first labour more out of accident than design. I arrived late at the hospital with my second labour out of deliberate design. I didn't want to go. My husband finally forced me into the car and we arrived there an hour before Pippa was born.

Apart from the episiotomy it was the normal, straightforward birth I had so much wanted but there was no euphoria, I felt too threatened. I asked to hold the baby and was given her, briefly, wrapped up tightly, her large eyes staring at me. I wanted to get up and take her home. This baby deserved a better atmosphere and greater joy at her birth. Her sister should have been with us to welcome her and we should all have been at home. Still, it could have been much worse, and for that I was grateful. I had reckoned without the postnatal wards.

It was like a prison camp up there. They were short-staffed and short-tempered. I was booked for forty-eight hours which turned into three days. I remember that time as a Kafkaesque nightmare with uniformed bullies deliberately confusing and tormenting me. I remember waking one morning to a heavy punch on the shoulder: 'Wake up. Your food's ready.' Every remark was snapped. 'Why are you in bed?', 'Why are you out of bed?', 'What are you doing out here?', 'What are you doing in there?' and even, amazingly, 'Don't talk while you're eating.' There was a rumpus one day when a mother called the sister a bitch. It was the only time I smiled.

In such an atmosphere I found it impossible to relate to the baby. I desperately missed Imogen who came to visit me but only wanted to ride up and down in the lift.

The paediatrician, a kind, overworked man, suspected that Pippa might be developing jaundice. He wanted me to stay in longer. Richard thought it would be wise. I felt desperate. That afternoon Richard and his mother came to visit me and the staff were rude to them as well. I collapsed in floods of tears. Richard went to collect my clothes and I was out in an hour. Pippa did not develop jaundice.

In terms of depression I was a low-risk mother when I had Imogen and a high-risk mother when I had Pippa. If I had not had witnesses to the unpleasantness in that ward I might have imagined I was being over-sensitive. But my mother-in-law who had been a nurse was horrified. I have no doubt that the staff were convinced I had baby blues.

The period immediately after birth is a time of great emotional vulnerability. Giving birth is such a sudden and dramatic event, it sweeps away emotional defences, it leaves us feeling raw and exposed both physically and emotionally:

> I think you're very vulnerable, ever so vulnerable. It's a bit of a tightrope, isn't it? You feel like you're going right across a very narrow path and you could fall off either side. You've got to get across. I think you know you're going to get there but if the wrong person's there at the wrong time, it can affect you.

This sums up very well the precarious position of the newly delivered mother as she meets and starts to care for her baby. Often the atmosphere in which she embarks on this task is far from helpful:

> Like the openness after you've had a baby, especially in hospital. I think it's a place that breeds neurosis because all the time they're testing and weighing, looking at motions and worried about being sterile and the whole thing.

As this woman points out, the starch, sterility and science are not exactly relaxing. The hospital controls the baby's routine and dictates when and for how long mothers can be with their babies. This upsets those mothers who want to be with their babies all the time but reassures mothers who feel worried about their ability to care for them.

Certainly high standards of cleanliness are essential in a hospital where there is always risk of cross-infection in nurseries. The main danger to babies, however, comes from highly resistant hospital germs, not the 'wild' germs brought in by the mother or her visitors. In the hospital I went to we were forbidden to put the baby on our own bed which was evidently regarded as a very dangerous place. Since we all bathed at least once a day, I never understood this rule.

The control of the baby's routine by the hospital is intended partly to give the mothers a chance to recover and partly to enable nurses to teach mothers basic baby care with a minimum of chaos. Some hospitals achieve this. All too often, however, the ward routine becomes an end in itself, an iron jacket into which all must fit: 'I got up into the ward at four a.m. and then they came along at six a.m. and woke me. I just had two hours' sleep.' The sheer madness of waking a woman who has just gone to sleep after being in labour all night is only matched by the equal insanity of waking women to see if they want sleeping pills! Nor is the training of mothers in baby care always very successful:

I didn't know how to feed him, I didn't know how to fold a nappy. I looked at the nappy and looked at his bottom and thought, 'Well I don't see how it fits.' I'd no idea. No one had actually ever shown me. I had to go to my doctor and ask him. He didn't know either, actually! They used disposables in the hospital and when they took him away to get him dressed I said, 'Well let me come and watch,' because I wanted to see how they did it and she said, 'Oh, no, you can't come, you've got to wait there.' It was all, you know, worked out, and so when I changed him for the first time I didn't know how to do it.

In part many of the complaints about postnatal wards arise because of staff shortages but in part they are also due to a basic antagonism between mothers and nurses. Ann Cartwright comments in her study *Human Relations and Hospital Care*[2] that maternity patients are less likely than others to feel grateful towards the hospital staff because they are not ill in the same way. They are also likely to be affected by the way the nurses look after their babies as well as the attention they personally receive. From the nurses' point of view, the maternity patients may evoke less sympathy because they are not ill and because their situation, with husbands and babies,

may seem enviable. Mothers may well appear more demanding and critical than other patients and the work itself is
relatively uninteresting with little variety and much mess.

Much of the job satisfaction in maternity nursing must
come from looking after the babies. This can create a situation of rivalry between mothers and nurses over who has
the baby. Mothers often feel that they are unable to be
close to their babies in hospital because the hospital staff
take charge of them and only permit a limited amount of
contact. Some nurses undoubtedly are envious and try to
displace the mother. Others dislike the work with inevitable
results:

> One girl came in and she said, 'I hate this bloody job, I
> hate these squalling kids!' This very funny Scottish girl
> said, 'Well, why the hell don't you get out of the job?' 'Oh,
> Christ there's nothing else to do!' I thought that one woman
> is making all these girls' lives a misery and she doesn't even
> like the job. Yet we have to put up with her and we are
> at our most vulnerable, our most sensitive. You feel
> so sensitive and . . . fragile is the word, fragile under-
> lined.

It is because of this emotional fragility that the kind of
care we receive in the days immediately after birth is so important. In order to be mothers to our babies we need mothering ourselves. It is a very private time this early period of
getting to know the baby. I remember watching a mother
freshly arrived from the labour ward in the bed next to me
being handed her baby to see. The nurse stood a few paces
away, arms folded, waiting to take the baby back to the
nursery. How could she be relaxed? It is like trying to make
love with the hotel maid stamping around outside waiting to
change the sheets.

With the best will in the world institutions cannot provide
the kind of cradling environment women need at this time.
That some come close to it is much to their credit. Many
don't even make the attempt.

Animal studies have shown that there is an important period
immediately after birth when the mother develops a bond

with her young. In his research with animals the Dutch zoologist Cornelius Naakteboren has noted the importance of licking. A ewe will reject her lamb if it is removed from her just after birth, dried with a towel and returned to her a few hours afterwards. Goats are even more extreme. If the kid is not kept with its mother for the first five minutes after delivery she will not become attached to it and will refuse to care for it, butting or kicking it away as it approaches her.

Human beings are infinitely more complex than animals. We can reason and use language. We are incredibly adaptable. Human behaviour is also a result more of learning than of instinct. If mothers, like those in Western countries, do not learn to breastfeed by watching other mothers, then they don't know how to do it. In view of this, maternal instinct, if it exists, has to be carefully defined. An instinct is biologically programmed. Fear produces instinctive responses; the muscles tense, adrenalin flows, breathing becomes quicker and the heart beats faster, sending blood to the muscles which are needed for a fast sprint out of danger. The body always reacts in this way whether fear is created by a charging bull in a field or a request to make a public speech. Unnecessary fear can be removed but the instinctive response to fear cannot.

If there is a maternal instinct it must have a stimulus and an invariable response. In the case of the sensitive period following birth it appears likely that there may be an instinctive response by undrugged mothers towards their young if they are allowed to see, hold and touch them immediately after birth. Klaus and Kennell filmed twelve mothers who were allowed maximum freedom in handling their naked newborn babies under a heat panel. They found an orderly and predictable pattern of behaviour; touching the hands and feet, caressing the body with the palms of the hands, increasing excitement and intense eye contact. Aidan Macfarlane, a British paediatrician, conducted similar research with slightly different results. He notes, however, that most of the babies in his sample were wrapped up and: 'The expression of deep emotions within our society very much depends on social custom. Childbirth is perhaps the one time when it is always acceptable to show emotion, but this still strongly depends on who is present to see and hear.'[3]

The importance of all this research lies in the fact that it supports the complaints that mothers have been making for years about the way hospitals interfere with their relationships with their babies. It helps mothers who desperately want to be close to their premature babies. It raises questions about the widespread use of drugs which leave both mother and baby doped at birth. It brings into focus the strangeness felt by mothers after Caesarean operations. It demands that more thought be given to the emotional environment surrounding women at birth.

Certainly we are so flexible as a species that we can compensate for an early loss of contact and certainly no mother should be forced through a ritual bonding period if she isn't initially interested in her baby. (God forbid that mother-and-baby bonding should ever become a timetabled hospital procedure!) But if an instinctive attachment between mother and baby is possible immediately after birth it *should* be positively worked for and encouraged in the most relaxed and informal way possible.

Frederick Leboyer, a French obstetrician, Dr Arthur Janov, an American psychologist, and R. D. Laing, the British psychiatrist, are all convinced that a traumatic birth with unnecessary separation of mother and baby leaves an indelible mark on the body and mind of the newborn baby. Leboyer says of traditional hospital birth:

Such is birth.

The torture of the innocent.

One would have to be naïve indeed to believe that so great a cataclysm would not leave its mark.

Its traces are everywhere; on the skin, in the bones, in the stomach, in the back, in all our human folly, in our madness, our tortures, our prisons, in legends, epics and in myths.[4]

We should be fortunate indeed if all our human folly and madness could so easily be eliminated at birth. Nonetheless, with a little imagination and empathy, the newborn child could be spared much suffering and her mother many tears.

Tears are very common in the postnatal wards. It has been variously estimated that between 50 per cent and 80 per cent of all mothers suffer from the third, fourth or tenth day blues. Irvin D. Yalom and his colleagues in Palo Alto, California, made a study of the post-partum blues syndrome and concluded that it 'is apparently self-limited and relatively benign'. They comment, however, on the great vulnerability of women in the first ten days after birth:

> Our clinical observations suggest that the most frequent experiential state of depressed mothers is one of great vulnerability. Regressive features are evident; the new mothers long to be cared for and to be mothered themselves. Any indication of personal slight or rejection precipitates transient depressive swings.[5]

Given this intense vulnerability, the average, busy, postnatal ward abounds with opportunities for new mothers to feel personal slight or rejection. The fact that tears are so common makes it easy to dismiss them as unimportant. Are they? In some cases yes, but in cases like this the misery is avoidable: 'I wanted to breastfeed but every nurse seemed to tell me something different. I tried for four days but gave up after that, feeling a failure and taking Valium.'

Whilst it is accepted that women cry a great deal for no very good reason after birth, it is rarely accepted that many women have good cause to cry:

> When Marie was seven days old my husband had been visiting and at 8.30 Marie started yelling. I let her yell for fifteen minutes, then I decided that everything I did wasn't going to settle her down so I started feeding her. I'd just got my baby settled on the breast when Sister —— came in and saw me feeding, so she just walked up and pulled Marie off the breast and tossed her back in the cot.[6]

If the mother were to burst into floods of tears after an incident like this, it would, probably, be interpreted as a fit of the blues caused by hormonal changes and oversensitivity.

In no research I have read concerning 'the blues' has there ever been a suggestion that the ward staff were anything but helpful and sympathetic. Tears like mine, shed as a result of humiliating treatment, are easily categorized as 'blues' and dismissed. They are not. They are signs of unhappiness due to ill-treatment. They should not be shed.

I was born at home in 1941. It was the middle of the black-out. Not a chink of light showed from any window in Britain to guide the Nazi bombers to their targets. I entered a land in darkness. I asked my mother what the midwife did with me after I was born. She said I had been washed and wrapped up warmly.

And then? My mother looked puzzled as though she did not quite understand the question. 'You were tucked up into bed with me of course.'

Of course.

7. 'I Remember, I Remember the House where I was Born'*

If having a baby in hospital can be such an upsetting experience, is a home birth any better? For a large number of women, yes. In her own home a woman's individual wishes matter, she is important. It is a private place for a private event, a family event.

> Eleanor was born at 12.10. She weighed 9 lb. 10 oz., but I didn't need an episiotomy . . . We all had a glass of elderflower wine which Wally had saved specially and I settled back with my parents and the *two* members of my own family, pleasantly warm with the first alcohol I had tasted for about nine months. I couldn't help wondering about my situation if I had been in hospital. There just is no comparison.[1]

In emotional terms there is no comparison. During the hospital strike early in 1973, sixty-five mothers in Ashton-under-Lyne were asked to have their babies at home instead of in hospital. A survey of these mothers published in *Midwife and Health Visitor*[2] showed that 90 per cent of mothers having their first baby would prefer to have their next at home. Seventy-two per cent of mothers who had their babies both in hospital and at home would prefer to have their next at home.

Some hospitals provide better emotional support than others but always the hospital is alien territory. There is no guarantee that the staff will be kind. This totally pointless suffering of a bad hospital experience as compared to home birth comes out in the following deeply disturbing account:

> I was still begging for gas and air but the sister was ushering her students in to watch the baby's head engaging with the comment: 'You may as well watch this.' I hated the

* 'Past and Present', Thomas Hood.

students being present but was at that time unable to protest. I was never at any time asked if I would mind if students watched the birth. I was delivered on my back – presumably because it was easier for the students to watch the delivery that way . . . As soon as the baby was born I heard the sister say, 'This is a premature infant' . . .

My husband told me we had a second daughter. I put my hands down for my baby and was given her – covered in vernix and very sweet. I had hardly put my arms around her when she was whisked away – to intensive care of course. The nurses all disappeared – I don't remember a kind word from any of them after the birth . . . No one has ever admitted that . . . I was induced prematurely.

I feel I have been physically and emotionally assaulted. I had severe postnatal depression and still cannot face a postnatal examination. I've no faith in doctors and I just don't want to be touched. I cannot get over the feeling that if I'd been a prize cow on a farm I might have been given better and kinder treatment.

I know that birth shouldn't be so traumatic. My second child's birth at home was a delight and thinking of it has helped me cope with my depression over this last birth.[3]

Again this woman directly connects her depression to a bad birth experience. It is the memory of a good birth which she feels has helped her.

If a good birth experience at home can help to reduce the numbers of women suffering from depression why are 97 per cent of all babies born in hospital? According to the Peel Report, published in 1970, hospital is the safest place for women to have babies; safest, that is, in terms of physical health. There has, as we might expect, been little research into which is safest in terms of mental health and how the risks balance out. Having a baby at home is, doctors argue, a very dangerous and risky business. The implication is that this has always been the case but now, thanks to the National Health, we can *all* have the advantages of hospital care denied to our mothers and grandmothers. Really?

My grandmother had ten children. All were born at home, delivered by the local midwife, Nurse Tyson, who used to ride round the villages on her bicycle and also attend to the children's teeth. All ten children survived infancy; one died of rheumatic fever at the age of ten and the other nine continued and continue into old age.

My grandmother was the wife of a farm labourer and could not possibly have afforded to pay for a doctor. This in itself served to protect her. At the turn of the century the traditional midwife carried a much lower risk of infection to her mothers than did doctors or doctor-controlled hospitals. These were the days when thousands of mothers died of puerperal fever, an infection caused by low standards of cleanliness on the part of those examining and delivering mothers. Still more mothers died as a result of medical over-enthusiasm for the use of forceps, a practice which Sir Frederick Truby King strongly attacked in 1922:

> Were the resorting to forced, rapid delivery through drugs, forceps and all such unnatural artificial processes restricted to the very small minority of cases in which their use is justifiable or beneficient, one might be sure there would result a rapid and welcome fall in our still-births, maternal deaths and deaths of babies at or about the time of birth.[4]

Such practices were not for the likes of my granny. They cost too much. Nor could my mother afford them; she delivered both her children at home. It was women who could afford the attendance of doctors with their full paraphernalia of drugs, forceps and general interference who were most at risk. In 1937 the British Ministry of Health produced a report which revealed that in 1930-2 in England and Wales maternal deaths were highest in social classes I and II. Puerperal sepsis (infection) was 20 per cent higher in social classes I and II than in social class V.[5] This report was published the year before my brother was born safely at home, delivered by the district midwife.

The move to hospital confinement has been one of the major changes for women in the past fifty years. In the 1920s only 15 per cent of all live births in Britain occurred in hospital. In 1976 only 3 per cent of babies were born at home. In consequence there has been a decline in the number of district midwives and a real struggle for mothers who want a home birth:

> We were unable to find a midwife, so my husband and I visited our GP. He would not examine me or even ask us to sit down. He totally opposed our wishes, said I was doing a very dangerous thing and that no doctor or midwife would attend me nor would he. We were made to feel like irresponsible idiots and were left in no doubt that a home confinement was totally forbidden.[6]

This kind of fierce reception by doctors to a request for a home confinement is by no means unusual, despite the fact that legally all women have a right to the choice of a home or hospital delivery. It is a choice which the vast majority of people in the community wish to retain. A recent Gallup poll conducted among 1054 people revealed that 82 per cent of women and 75 per cent of men agree that facilities for home births should be made available.[7]

The government officially supports a move to 100 per cent hospital confinements as does the Royal College of Midwives and most doctors. There is a clear conflict between the wishes of the community and the opinion of professionals supported by government. This conflict has turned the home births issue into a political fight. Answering a parliamentary question from the Tory health spokesman Patrick Jenkin in spring 1978 Mr David Ennals, then Secretary of State for Social Services, said that if a woman opted for home delivery despite arguments against it, health authorities should ensure that the services necessary to make home delivery as safe as possible are provided. It is to be hoped that these are not pious words: there are parts of the country where these services have been phased out already.

In 1975 Newcastle Area Health Authority put out a document entitled 'Procedure for Requesting a Home Confinement' which stated that 'the present practice of obstetrics no longer makes it a satisfactory procedure for a midwife to accept a patient for home confinement . . . one would be extremely critical of any midwife who took this action and she may well find herself in the position of having a case of malpractice to answer . . .'[8] The Newcastle Area Health Authority has thus achieved the distinction of having more babies born in ambulances than at home.

The case against home deliveries is difficult to prove. Where emergency back-up services are available, home deliveries are remarkably safe for the healthy, low-risk mother. Holland has a lower death rate than Britain and 50 per cent of Dutch babies are born at home. America for all its technology, drugs and complete medical control has more infant deaths a year than fifteen other 'civilized' countries. Nor is 'uncivilized' birth always as dangerous as we may imagine. A study of childbirth among Punjab village women in the 1960s discovered that where a leather worker's knife was used to cut the umbilical cord (as opposed to scissors) the death rate for babies was 27 per thousand, the equivalent of British infant death rates in 1953.[9]

There is a direct relationship between poverty, poor nutrition, poor antenatal care and high infant death rates. The dramatic decline in infant mortality in Britain was closely connected with an improved standard of living, general public health measures and contraception. Healthy women living in healthy conditions with control of their fertility will produce more healthy live babies. In Britain today low-income women are high-risk mothers which is why good antenatal care is so important. The same is true of America, but there the expensive private medical system ensures that few poor women can afford antenatal care. The Scandinavian countries, on the other hand, where incomes are more evenly spread, provide thorough antenatal care, and have fewer babies dying at birth. In other words it is good food and good antenatal care which reduce the risks of stillbirth, not the routine use of birth technology.

So how dangerous *is* home birth? Certainly there are risks of unforeseen complications arising, which is why emergency back-up services are needed. No birth is entirely free of risk wherever it takes place. Avoidable infant deaths take place in hospital as well as at home. A district midwife has a limited amount of equipment but concentrates exclusively on one birth at a time. The hospital midwife has a great deal of equipment but is looking after a number of women. With a sudden delivery this has its dangers:

> I had a precipitate delivery in the bed at half past one in the morning; there was this black thing that I thought was dead. He was 2½ lb. It was obviously very traumatic. They resuscitated him in the bed, I heard him cry, but it was a long time before I could believe he was alive. There were people milling around but I don't think anybody realized quite how far on I was.

Assessing the risk in real figures, one study of stillbirths shows that during the period 1969-73 the stillbirth rate for home confinements was 4.5 per 1000 births,[10] a very low figure indeed, as it should be.

Compared to this risk, what are the risks of depression following a hospital delivery? What evidence there is, and once again there isn't much, suggests that more mothers get depressed following a hospital birth than a home birth. In one study of Cardiff mothers giving birth at home or in hospital in 1969-70 it was found that 64 per cent of the 107 women delivered in hospital experienced depression, compared with 19 per cent of the 86 women delivered at home.[11] A plea was made for further study to explain the difference. There has been none. Further evidence might be found, however, by comparing the low rates of depression in two studies carried out in general practice with the high rates of depression in two studies carried out in maternity units. The general practice studies showed incidence of depression requiring treatment of 2.8 per cent[12] and 3 per cent[13] out of samples of 700 and 313 respectively. The hospital studies on the other hand showed rates of 10.8 per cent [14] and 7 per cent[15] out of samples of 305 and 189 respectively.

It can be argued that the difference in the figures could be due, in part at least, to the number of home births in the general practice samples. Unfortunately neither of the studies differentiates between home and hospital births but any sample taken from general practice in the early 1960s would probably have a fairly high proportion of home births. The national average for home confinements in the early 1960s was 40 per cent. Of course regions varied.

Certainly there are a number of psychiatrists who have linked hospital deliveries with emotional disturbance. In *Modern Perspectives in Psycho-obstetrics* is the strong statement that: 'There is little doubt that the incidence of puerperal depression, of emotional disorder generally, and of disturbances in the mother-baby relationship, are less frequent in home confinements than in hospital confinements.'[16] And in *Psychiatric Disorders in Obstetrics* there is a similar statement: 'Major psychoses develop very much more frequently in mothers delivered in a maternity unit than in mothers delivered at home.'

There is a further statement that: 'Four day blues . . . is more common following hospital confinement than at home.'[17] Dr Elizabeth Tylden of University College Hospital, London, also states that severe mental depression is found almost exclusively in women who have their babies in hospital.[18]

Since there is no connection between postnatal depression and physical complications in labour the reason why more mothers are miserable in hospital than at home must be connected to the way they are treated there. Dr Bardon has written:

It should certainly be a matter for professional debate as to how accurately the physical risks of home confinement can be weighed against the psychological risks to the mother-child relationship of hospital confinement in an unfavourable setting. This debate cannot usefully occur in the absence of those paediatricians and psychologists who have made careful objective studies of mother-neonate interactions.[19]

Certainly there should be a professional debate if the specialists can bring themselves to talk to each other. In the meantime women are judging for themselves and doggedly insisting on their right to give birth at home.

Needless to say we are not warned about the emotional dangers of having a baby in hospital. Trust is the name of the game, complete trust and confidence in the experts – all six, eight, ten or more of them! Most of the women who fight to have their babies at home do so because they feel that birth is a natural event, a family event; because they want their own space around them; they want to be with familiar faces, husbands, children, parents, friends – and the midwife.

The midwife who attends a home birth is a very important figure; she is female, familiar, experienced and patient. The Newsons comment in their study on infant care[20] that however busy the midwife may be she always seems able to provide the real friendliness and intimacy which is a great support to women in labour and which is often lacking in an institution.

District midwives, for all their heavy workload are less bossy and harassed than hospital midwives. They know their mothers. They are independent practitioners; they do not have to conform to routine procedures like episiotomy. They have the judgement and confidence that comes from experience. The following account of a labour considered to have had complications pays tribute to the skills of the experienced district midwife; skills which may soon be lost both to us and our daughters:

> My little girl was born five minutes later – eyes wide open, gazing quietly round the room. We hadn't even made up the bed properly. So why am I writing all this? Perhaps it is because I have more faith in a midwife's experience; twenty-five years in the district, and over 2000 births attended, than perhaps a younger houseman's ability to read information pushed out by machines. Why did I stay at home? To have someone familiar at the bottom of the bed, and to avoid having another devastating episiotomy.[21]

In 1962, when 40 per cent of all births were home confinements and there were not enough hospital beds available for mothers who wanted them, a book by Claire Rayner was published called *Mothers and Midwives*. In this book she investigates conditions and complaints by both mothers and midwives about hospital and home birth. It is a depressing fact that all the complaints about hospitals which she looked at sixteen years ago are still pouring in: bad communications, callousness, being left alone in labour and babies separated

from mothers after birth. Added to this list are now the complaints about the active management of labour and the difficulty of booking a home confinement.

In the very different political climate which surrounded
home confinements in 1962 she comments: 'When one looks
dispassionately at the whole picture, the mystery is not that
the district-delivered mothers have so few complaints to
make, but that so many women still demand hospital confinement.'[22]

Health is more than the absence of symptoms. A healthy
young woman who fights to have her baby at home is assert-
ing her belief in a natural process; her faith in her body; her
rejection of the medicalization of birth. She is healthy. Her
fight is healthy.

Ivan Illich, the controversial philosopher, has written about
the dangers to health of the medicalization of life. He calls
this 'social iatrogenesis' (doctor-created illness). He says:

Social iatrogenesis is at work when health care is turned
into a standardized item, a staple; when all suffering is
'hospitalized' and homes become inhospitable to birth,
sickness and death; when the language in which people
could experience their bodies is turned into bureaucratic
gobbledegook; or when suffering, mourning and healing
outside the patient role are labelled a form of deviance.[23]

Birth-as-illness is already with us and women are labelled
as deviants who seek to give birth without hospital, drugs
or interference. The language of obstetrics alienates us from
our own bodies and makes us afraid. We become bemused
spectators at the births of our own children.

Birth and death are the two great mysteries of our human
condition. Both have been 'hospitalized', shrouded in a professional mystique and removed from the community. Nor can
we entirely blame doctors for conspiring to achieve this. We
are all to blame in that we have handed over to them the
responsibility for our pain, our worry, our grief. We expect
that, like priests, they will know how to soothe our sore and
jangled spirits. It is a heavy burden for them to carry and

not one for which they are equipped by training. We are now so protected from the major dramas of life: birth, insanity, physical suffering and death that we have lost the ability to cope with them. We are afraid. We have no accepted rituals, no communal resources to help us. In the name of science and objectivity we have dismantled a folk culture which could have supported our suffering, shared our joy. In its place we have drugs, hospitals and a wasteland of loneliness.

Birth is good. It is exciting, it is human; it brings joy to the jaded and new hope for the future. It belongs to us all. It reflects and affects our experience. Birth has its risks, its tragedies, its bitterness; it carries the ambivalence of all human experience but it is not and never will be an illness.

8. *Father's Day*

What about fathers? No one, needless to say, bothers themselves overmuch about how a man feels about becoming a
father. A shadowy figure, influential but ill-defined, he hovers
around somewhere behind the mother. If he is married it is
assumed he will shoulder his responsibilities and support his
wife financially and emotionally; if he is unmarried it is
assumed he will do the opposite.

Dulan Barber has commented in his book on unmarried
fathers: 'Little is known, said or written about unmarried
fathers because society expects them to remove themselves,
even to run away from the situation they have helped to
create . . . Society offers no other model to the unmarried
father and certainly does not take into consideration his
feelings and problems.'[1] Nor does society take into consideration the feelings and problems of the married father or,
come to that, the step-father, adoptive father, foster father
or divorced father. Fatherhood is simply not regarded as being very important to men. There are thousands upon thousands of books written by men about motherhood but a bare
handful by men about fatherhood.

Children belong to women, they are the mother's responsibility and are not expected to have much effect on their
father. A man's involvement must be with his work in the
outside world. A National Union of Journalists bulletin
describes how members in one organization were pressing
for a crèche. The management pointed out that there were
few women workers. They were told, however, that there were
plenty of men, many of them fathers. The puzzled management
said, 'You mean it would be used by men's wives' children?'[2]
The bemused rejection of the responsibilities of fatherhood
by the management of this organization is only noteworthy
because of the language they chose to use. Other manage-
ments have exactly the same views but don't talk so revealingly about 'men's wives' children'.

A man does not expect and is not expected to adapt his life to the arrival of children. He will continue with his work and his leisure pursuits and to a greater or lesser degree take an active interest in his children's development. It is the wife who will give up paid employment to be responsible for the children and the home. This division of responsibilities is so traditional it usually isn't even discussed: 'I was the one who said, "now is the time". I mean my husband had always said, "You know that I want children but you will have to make the sacrifices, therefore you decide the time," although I don't think it was even verbalized to that extent.'

Despite the fact that he needs to make less obvious social adjustment, the father nonetheless has to cope with considerable emotional adjustment. He too has his resentment and must do something with it. He may direct it at himself, he may try to obliterate it with his mates in the pub, he may direct it at his wife, feeling the baby has replaced him in her affections. Books written for the expectant mother often end with a cheery encouragement not to make her husband feel out of it: 'But remember that your husband has been deprived of your company for a long time and see to it that the new member of the family does not mean that he has less of your love, time and affection.'⁸ Well meaning, no doubt, but hopelessly impractical when you consider the enormous emotional upheaval in a marriage following the birth of a baby. It also implies that child and father are locked in deadly rivalry for the mother's love, time and affection which may indeed be true, but if she sees herself as living to satisfy rival claims she will end up negating herself and being of little use to either.

The birth of a baby represents a crisis for the entire family, including the father. In the past, when families were larger and marriages less intimate, the patriarchal father could remain aloof from the whole business. Marriage and the family were important as institutions because they controlled sexuality and guaranteed paternity. Legitimate sons would inherit property, titles and the family name. The attitudes displayed by society towards unmarried mothers showed quite clearly that only legitimate children mattered. These attitudes are still with us today, despite the dramatic social changes which have occurred this century.

Because men are economically and socially more privileged than women, attempts to adjust their role are seen as threats. Men learn to equate their superiority over women with virility. A building-site mentality towards women is encouraged in the name of manliness. Rape and wife beating are logical results of this equation and women who refuse to submit to domination are accused of 'provoking' both. Violence against women is masculine and who can sensibly accuse a man of being over-virile? Man's inhumanity to woman is so deeply etched into our culture that it is generally assumed to be biologically determined. Men, we are told, are 'naturally' more aggressive than women and less capable of controlling their violence or lust. The fact that their violence may land them in the law courts creates for men a double bind of heads-I-win-tails-you-lose situation: to be non-violent is 'cissy'; to be violent is criminal.

Fortunately most men manage to live with this contradiction without inflicting too much physical or verbal violence on women. Nonetheless the threat is there. Women have to live with the fact that our society expects men to control them, by violence if necessary.

This centuries-old assumption that a man must control his family is reinforced by law and custom. Married women are defined as 'dependants' by the state and custom dictates that they should change their name on marriage. Yet the position of women has changed. Married women have developed a taste for economic independence and increasingly reject the corset of their traditional role. Men, too, have to change but they are not helped to do this:

In our rapidly changing society, men and women are searching for new roles. What they seek might be expressed as: 'Women must work and men must weep.' Society partially supports the woman in her quest, but the man hardly at all.

If a man wants to weep, to develop his sensitivity, to express his emotions, his virility, maturity and strength are all called in question.[4]

So writes Ruth Forbes, magistrate and antenatal teacher, in a paper on the father's role. She recognizes that the birth of a child is a time of emotional stress for fathers which their traditional role denies.

If the state of marriage were simply a matter of performing social roles (breadwinner/housewife) then men would find no problems in this situation. Marriage, however, is very much more than a social institution, it is an interdependent love relationship between two people, and when a child is born both have to make emotional adjustments. Because a man doesn't expect to, he may be taken completely unawares, as this father discovered:

> I suspected that they would take up a lot of time but I didn't think there would be so much hard graft. I suspected, for example, that it would trap me in a marriage more than the marriage with a piece of paper did, previously, but I really didn't account for the emotional reaction that that entrapment brought with it. The biggest thing is the almost sense of despair that you can no longer think of yourself as emotionally free. To a certain extent you can think of yourself as emotionally free from your wife, but when it's your own flesh and blood, that emotional bond with the child is as negative as it is positive and in that way it rips you apart.

There is also the fact that once a man becomes a father, he is a breadwinner with a vengeance. Gone are the dreams of throwing it all in and starting up a business of his own. Gone are the moments when he could tell the boss where to stuff his bloody job. He has dependants, he is no longer debonair and fancy free. One reaction to this is to have an affair while his wife is pregnant. By doing this he will be breaking free in the traditional way expected of young males. It is partly a response to the feeling of responsibilities to come (much like a stag party). There may in addition be sexual rejection from his wife, who can't face intercourse with a bump, and certainly there will be some feeling of the old taboos about sex during pregnancy. He will also be receiving from a mistress some attention for himself instead of having to give attention to his wife.

It is not easy for men to communicate the anxieties they feel when their wives are pregnant. The spotlight is on the woman who is experiencing physical changes, often discomfort and who requires support. She receives the attention of doctors, midwives, friends and relatives and he picks up what information there is by the way. He is not supposed to appear too interested in this 'woman's business'. In all probability he is totally ignorant about the whole process of birth, thinking of it in terms of blood and pain and possibly experiencing some envy.

Isolated within the nuclear family with a work role which allows for little expression of feeling, all too many men turn to their accepted outlets to relieve the tension and confusion which they feel: booze, extra-marital sex, overwork and the sportsfield. All these are activities which take them away from the home and leave the wife feeling abandoned and resentful.

An alternative to these traditional outlets is to become involved in the pregnancy by attending antenatal classes and learning about birth. The father who does this can be a tremendous source of support to his wife during labour. He will also be involved in rather than excluded from the experience of his child's birth.

Research conducted at Charing Cross Hospital following antenatal instruction of both husband and wife showed that of the 730 husbands questioned 61.3 per cent were present for the whole labour of whom 99.6 per cent were glad they were present and only 0.2 per cent regretted it. There was a strong social bias to the upper groups.[5]

The class difference in this survey probably reflects the more traditional attitudes of working-class men, at least in their public image. A hospital confinement is a public affair. In the days of home confinements the working-class father was often with his wife during labour even if he didn't actually attend the delivery.

Apart from providing emotional support for his wife during labour, a husband can also protect her from any frightening procedures or callous treatment. It is much easier for him to do this if he knows it might be necessary because hospitals can intimidate husbands too. Hospitals recognize the presence of the husband as a potential threat to their authority and some of the worst ones apparently welcome husbands but do everything possible to persuade them to go home once they have arrived.

It has taken a great deal of pressure to persuade hospitals to allow fathers to be present at the birth of their children and many still see them as intruders. One woman I knew who insisted foetal monitoring machines be disconnected because she could not tolerate them was badgered by no fewer than twelve different people to persuade her to change her mind. Only a determined and strong-willed husband protected her from all that pressure. She gave birth to a healthy baby.

To witness the emergence of one body from another, which is birth, is a breathtaking event. It would be surprising if fathers weren't moved by it and most are:

I think they get in a terrible state because a friend of mine had a baby five weeks after me and the first thing her husband did was to come round to me and have breakfast at some unearthly hour in the morning and just talk about this baby and how he felt. I'd never talked to him like that before at all. I suppose he thought I'd understand. He felt completely confused really, excited that he was there all the time while the baby was born. He went through the whole thing. It was quite amazing and he's a very shy person you know. Being at the birth was obviously enormously important.

Even fathers who have never intended to be present can become completely absorbed by the experience:

Mine wasn't going to be there and then he got stuck between the oxygen bottle and the bed and they completely forgot about him and he sort of stayed there, terrified. He knew a *bit* about it, because I'd told him a *bit*. He said the first thing he noticed was the imprint on the soles of the baby's feet. He couldn't get over that, that there should actually be feet like we've got. That was the thing that struck him most.

There is a general belief that fathers who have been present at the birth of their babies are likely to be more involved with them afterwards:

> I think it does make a difference though, you know, talking to husbands or fathers that haven't been present at the birth there seems to be a . . . I don't know . . . less identification somehow, less of a feeling that it's yours.

This observation is supported by a study in Sweden where a group of fathers who had been asked to undress their babies twice within the first five days of life were compared with a group of fathers who did not have that experience. There was a significant difference in the amount of time the fathers spent playing with their babies three months later if they had had that early experience.[6]

However, a professor of psychology can write: 'There is, for that matter, no reason why the mothering role should not be filled as competently by males as females. The human male's relative lack of involvement in child rearing is essentially a cultural rather than a biological phenomenon.'[7] Just let him try presenting that case down at the social security office! A widower who feels that he can care better for his children in their grief than a strange woman, is likely to be regarded as a skyver and pressured into getting a job.

The law is no more sympathetic. A twenty-one-year-old student teacher who had postponed his training to stay at home and look after his baby lost his custody case despite evidence which showed that he had done a good job of dealing with the child's needs without assistance. The President of the Family Division at the Magistrates Court commented on his case: 'There is, I think, in the minds of most people something not very satisfactory in the idea of a young man *giving up all* [my italics] to look after a baby when there is a mother willing and able to do so.'[8] In other words why sweep the floor when there's a servant to do it? The student lost custody of his baby because the court considered caring for a child too trivial and unimportant a matter for a man.

We all know that children need consistent loving care in order to grow and develop fully. We live in a society where the giving of that care is regarded as an inferior job to be done by people who have nothing better to contribute. This conflict between the high intrinsic value of child care and its low social status has serious consequences for women and children. It also affects men, most particularly those men who want to be loving and involved fathers.

If his wife will tolerate it, and many women have no choice, a man can, with impunity, content himself with simply being a biological father and take no further interest in his children. In one study of the social situation of women, Professor D. R. Miller of the School of Social Sciences at Brunel University concludes:

> In reviewing these results one is impressed by the success with which so many groups of middle-aged women have been socialized to live amicably in a Victorian society where men control the marital relationship and favour the company of their mates in the pub or club. Not surprisingly, it is these women, who would rather have sons than daughters, who are inclined to denigrate themselves and are cold in their sexual relations. Judging from the very different values of young bureaucratic women in the cities, the Victorian form of socialization will be as dead as the Dodo in another generation.[9]

If he is correct, and I can't entirely share his confidence, then the pressure on men to adapt their role will be even greater than it is at the moment. In Russia where women are much more emancipated and where men have, apparently, failed to adjust, one in three of all marriages ends in divorce and the average family in towns is one child. Soviet sociologists have established that two-thirds to three-quarters of all divorces are initiated by women. Soviet leaders are worried by the low birth rate.[10] We might speculate from this that women who are financially self-supporting will not tolerate husbands who leave them holding the baby and doing all the washing up.

Many fathers suffer already from these conflicting pressures. Society expects them to be aggressive and carve their way into the world; their wives expect them to provide emotional support and be involved in the care of the children. A few men can cope with both but for most the birth of a baby is a time of anxiety and confusion. Fortunately wives appreciate the problems:

> I think this is because of the family business, it's broken up now and people live on their own. You used to have Mums and Dads and aunties or *someone* round the corner and now the husband is really the only sort of beating post. Of course you expect him to be everything from father to lover to housekeeper to Evelyn Home to everything. Well, I mean, I was like that and I realize now that it was a huge mistake and for both of us it was quite a shock.

It is quite a shock, and men need support too: 'I think it's a rotten time for men actually because they've got to tell everybody and be on their own. Then mother-in-law might arrive and all they want to do is to talk to their wife and take the baby home.'

While the baby needs feeding during the night a wife will be exhausted and emotionally vulnerable. She probably won't feel much like sex, especially if she has had an episiotomy. Everything is disjointed in these early days and marriages easily deteriorate.

There is nothing in the traditional male role which helps a man to cope with the nurturing his wife needs whilst she is nurturing their baby. Men expect to receive care, not to give it:

> Well, he was terrified. He couldn't handle me, he couldn't handle the baby. He was terrified of the baby, didn't know what to *do* about it, didn't know how to hold it. I expected lots from him that I didn't get so therefore we had this sort of triangle which didn't resolve itself for a long time. I

think if I'd had parents or relations or somebody, it wouldn't have been so bad. I could have gone to see them and just sort of got all my frustrations and worries out before he came home and I immediately opened the door saying 'YOU'RE LATE! WHERE'VE YOU BEEN? WHAT'VE YOU BEEN DOING?' I mean the classic sort of awful wife. I cringe when I think about it now. I think one expects an awful lot from the husband that he simply cannot give. I expected a lot of help and support which I did get but not the kind I thought I'd get. I got practical things like cleaning the floor, doing the shopping, which was marvellous, but it wasn't what I wanted which was sort of understanding.

This last comment highlights the problem which men have in providing emotional support. They are good at *doing* things not at *being* understanding. They offer practical solutions but when comfort and care are required it is as though they seize up. This process is described very well by the following woman: 'He just translates any pain I have into his pain and I suppose that's a male thing. I am no longer the one with a problem and he's doubled his problems.'[11] It is a process which does not help anyone since it makes the man feel bad, without in any way helping the woman. Empathy means the ability to identify emotionally with another person and imaginatively enter their experience whilst still retaining a sense of self. It is not a quality encouraged in men.

Unless the lines of communication are kept open it is very easy for resentment to build up on each side. He thinks he is doing his best and working hard all day and resents coming home to a miserable and bad-tempered wife, who ought to pull herself together. She feels that he takes her for granted and simply will not see how much she has to do and how radically her life has altered.

When the baby was two months old he got a job which was very different from the job he'd had before. He was totally involved in it. He was meeting a lot of interesting people which meant that there was a terrific temptation on his part to go to the pub with them after work rather than coming home. So I felt the traditional wife's neglect and was furious. I was just furious. In fact it was he that said to me, 'For Christ's sake go back to work!' because our rows about him not coming home, in fact about everything were increasing. It was resentment and frustration. I had got to the stage where I felt very confined, particularly since I was looking after a friend's baby as well which meant that even going for a walk was a fairly major undertaking.

Or she feels resentful that he isn't helping as much as he might, that he is not prepared to change his life and be involved with the baby:

With me it was definitely that I didn't feel as though he was pulling his weight. That was the basic thing. Because I felt so harassed by the whole thing; this *thing* I had to look after 100 per cent of the time. I really didn't feel he did enough, even bearing in mind the fact that he was working and so on because I think that even when the wife works she's still expected to do everything at home as well, or I was anyway.

It is ironic that marriage, supposedly instituted for the procreation of children is most threatened after the birth of a baby. If the community fails to support the new family during these early months then it is in danger. The effect of this on the mother is obvious, not only does she feel alone and vulnerable but she sees her marriage disintegrating too. It is another piece in that stained glass window.

Theoretically husbands are in the best position to notice if their wives are becoming depressed, yet few do. Of all the women I have spoken to who have suffered from postnatal depression, only one had a husband who found help for her. She was a woman who became convinced that the baby was dead and she was dying, a psychotic reaction so dramatic it could scarcely be missed.

There was a joke I heard once which ran as follows:

Wife: I'm wearing something I haven't worn for over thirty years, haven't you noticed?

Husband: Em . . . very nice dress dear.

Wife: It's not the dress.

Husband: Oh . . . the shoes?

Wife: It's not the shoes.

Husband: I don't know!

Wife: I'm wearing my old gas mask from the war.

Husbands are not very observant. Habit and familiarity blunt the edges of awareness. Depression can be a slow quicksand and a man preoccupied with his own problems can easily fail to notice what is happening. Even if he does notice, he is more likely to blame his wife for being miserable and bad tempered than to consider that she needs help. After all, she's got the baby she wanted, what's she so miserable about?

I have often noticed that husbands will try to shrug off the problems that their wives have been through, as though it were too uncomfortable to admit that depression could strike so close to home. Most men, anyway, know very little about postnatal depression and it is not easy to live with a person who is totally absorbed in her own despair. Perhaps if husbands were more aware of the problem they would behave better. A few manage to cope incredibly well: 'Bill just took over completely, he did everything. He looked after the baby and he looked after the house and fed me. I just went off somewhere to sleep more or less. I can't remember very much. From when I was given the drugs there's sort of a blank. I was only seventeen and he was twenty-two.'

Too many, though, are plain bloody insensitive:

Then I started to get a bit tearful and one night my husband said, 'Oh for goodness sake pull yourself together! I'm going to ring the doctor. You know where she'll send you!' – we've got this enormous mental hospital that towers over the town – I said, 'Oh no, don't ring her!' He said, 'That's where she'll send you!' And so, of course, after that, everything was bottled up. I knew I couldn't cry in front of him or say anything to him. It was all 'Pull yourself together. It's ridiculous. People have four children and manage to cope. What's the matter with you, you ought to be able to cope.' He didn't show any sympathy at all. I think this was the big thing. If a husband can show sympathy it must make a difference.

9. Margaret's Story

'I know exactly why I was depressed. I mean I've got no problems about it now really except that nobody helped.

'My husband left to take up this new job which was very demanding, very stressful, when she was about ten days old. I packed up because I thought I was this great, strong female and I had a seventeen-month-old and this brand new baby. Well, obviously, I was absolutely knackered. I mean, I packed, I did all the packing and I shifted all the furniture and God knows what. It was absolutely stupid.

'Then when we moved, not surprisingly, I had no milk and nobody to consult. I didn't manage to build up the milk supply, Sarah cried constantly. I know now that she was hungry all the time of course. We were very isolated, right on the edge of the moors, which for someone who'd got used to living in London was pretty bleak.

'It was two and a half miles to the shops and two and a half miles back and I had Ben on the pram seat. There were perfectly good reasons to be depressed. But it lasted until she was nine months old and I didn't know what was happening to me then. I didn't know why I was always crying when my husband came home. Always there'd be Sarah and me crying and poor Ben all worried. My husband had enough problems with trying to make a new job work, a bit different to London, everything so different to London.

'A sympathetic GP could have said, "Well, there's a, b, c," you know? It could have been really easy for anyone outside. I mean I didn't have any friends, didn't know anyone . . . if I'd managed to make some friends . . . but the trouble is . . . when I was depressed I was very much locked inside myself and the kids . . .

'GPs are pretty ignorant aren't they? Depression's a tricky thing for them to deal with, they don't know much about it, they're too overburdened to go on refresher courses they ought to go on. I went to this GP just after we moved. He said,

"You've been reading things like *Reader's Digest* haven't you?" and I was very hurt. I was so low. I came down the surgery steps in tears. It was awful, he was horrible, I *never* forgot that. I mean I said, "I think I'm depressed" or something and therefore I had attempted self-diagnosis which is not allowed, it means that you've been reading things like *Reader's Digest*.

'If he'd looked at my medical notes he'd have seen that I'd had problems before the birth. My haemoglobin was low, I needed iron, I'm sure I did. It was almost, not quite, as simple as that, but that was one thing, one positive thing he could have done for me.

'When I went to this bloke it was when I'd thrown Sarah on the mat and I thought I'd broken her arm because she was about three months. I just sort of had this mental image of the headlines that were going to be in the paper . . . I'd picked her up like this and threw her . . . and what did he do? He told me I'd been reading *Reader's Digest*!

'Now it's so bloody straightforward and so damned frustrating because Sarah and I lost something that we've just begun to make up. I mean it took me a long time to like Sarah. And Ben spent so much time being good and he was only a baby. He wasn't even old enough for a playgroup or anything. He spent all his time being good because I was saying "I'm just busy with Sarah" and she would scream and scream and scream. We used to shut her in the little bedroom and go up to the end of the garden which was right on the moors and play games. But both of us, I'm sure, could hear her crying in our heads, even if we couldn't hear her crying. So he lost out because he was being good all the time, very consciously being a good baby who could help me because he loved me. And poor Sarah missed out because she spent nine months screaming because her mother was so cross and so miserable with her and also she was starving . . . She's OK now but I very much resent that GP and I would never, ever forgive the bloke for not . . . OK so I was new on the books, all right, I'd come from London – so what?

'We didn't even have a proper health visitor you see. We just had a mobile caravan that came, a little tiny caravan, you know how cramped they are? I only went for her injections, so nobody ever came to call at the house, or there might have been some help there. I know that these doctors here would have been much nicer, if we'd been living here instead of where we were.

'I was just bloody unlucky, but there are too many people who are just bloody unlucky like that aren't there? I shall never forget how I felt when I thought I'd broken her arm.

'I feel nothing but resentment, not at other people necessarily but just for moving, at us for being so silly. Why did he go away when Sarah was ten days old? Why on earth did I pack up the house? There were lots of friends offering to help. Why did I have to be so clever and shift wardrobes on my own and fill packing cases, who the hell did *I* think I was! I'm angry at myself mostly about it, trying to be too capable. I'm somebody who likes to manage everything by myself which is why I did it. "I can manage," I said with a seventeen-month-old and a ten-day-old, "I can pack up the flat and move us" – how stupid! Superwoman, Christ, some bloody superwoman I turned out! I'm very angry at myself. I wouldn't do it again, nor would I let anyone else do it.

'There was such a difference being the mother of one beautiful child in trendy London and being the mother of two on the edge of the Yorkshire moors where we knew nobody. That was what was wrong, I suppose, not having friends. I think *the* worst thing people can do is move at that time. I didn't need hospitalization or anything like that but I was bloody miserable for a hell of a long time and so weary and horrible to live with. It was just a horrible year, an awful year, a really wasted one.'

10. *Cabbage Days*

Some discouragement, some faintness of heart at the new real future which replaces the imaginary, is not unusual, and we do not expect people to be deeply moved by what is not unusual. That element of tragedy which lies in the very fact of frequency, has not yet wrought itself into the coarse emotion of mankind; and perhaps our frames could hardly bear much of it. If we had a keen vision and feeling of all ordinary human life, i‘ would be like hearing the grass grow and the squirrel's heart beat, and we should die of that roar which lies on the other side of silence. As it is, the quickest of us walk about well wadded with stupidity.

Middlemarch, George Eliot

The problems of the housebound mother are a part of 'that element of tragedy which lies in the very fact of frequency'. There is nothing so very unusual about the difficulties which women encounter when they arrive home with a new baby. We are not moved to anger or pity by the image of a tired mother alone with a screaming baby. It is too domestic and familiar, too common and undramatic to excite our interest. Only when the tired, isolated mother attacks herself or the baby do we perceive that element of tragedy:

My second screamed solidly for the first month, all through the nights, and slept in the day and nothing I could do would break this cycle and, of course, I had a toddler who did the opposite. So everybody else got some sleep except me. I can remember going to the doctor and saying that she was crying all the time and the doctor said, 'Well, I expect it's this three-month colic thing they get. It'll stop, three months and it'll see the end of it,' and it was as if she'd hit me in the face. I sat there and thought, 'Three months! I don't know how to get through till tomorrow morning!'

Three months could have been three years. I walked out pushing the pram and went home and dealt with them all: fed my husband, fed Andrew and got him to bed, gave the baby her feed and put her to bed and walked off.

We were living in a tiny little rural part of Wales, delightful place to live except when you're depressed. I walked and stood on the bridge over the river and was quite determined to drown myself, but every time I reached the point of thinking 'Here we go!' I just thought of the two of them and couldn't do it. But I *wanted* to do it, you see, this is the dreadful, dreadful thing, that I *wanted* to do it.

We do not know how many women come close to death in this way, nor how many just avoid damaging their children. We don't care to think of these things; they belong to the roar which lies on the other side of silence.

The stresses which form that mountain of sand deposited outside the home of each new mother are intricate and inter-related. Mothering the baby is 'natural' and therefore receives no recognition. Mother is not an occupational category, housewife is. The mother-housewife earns no money and therefore has no status. She does not 'work' but functions alone in her own home. Lack of recognition and repetitive work lead to feelings of fragmentation; exhaustion reinforces isolation; isolation and low status compound to create feelings of worthlessness.

Considering the sheer weight and pressure of all those grains of sand, the surprising thing is not that many women become pressed down by it all but that most do not. The framework which our society provides for mothers rearing their young is cramped, hostile and disordered:

It's this whole difference between the carrot that society feeds pregnant women, this image of the rosy-glow BMA-publication-type lady who's floating along in a filmy dress and then – wow, she comes out the other side and nobody wants to know her. You can't go into cafés because your baby will scream; you can't get your pram into shops but if you leave it outside you're doing the wrong thing; if you stop at home you're doing the wrong thing; you can't get help on buses; you can't go and see friends or it'll be sick on the carpet. You can't do *anything* and it *all* changes. Just nobody loves you do they?

No one bothers too much about the problems of the new mother because of the common belief that looking after babies is instinctive and not skilled. This leads easily to feelings of failure. If women, supposedly, have a biological instinct which enables them to know how to feed, comfort and care for their young, then the woman who doesn't know where to begin and may not even like her baby very much is unsexed. No one in this position is likely to admit to having problems or to seek help for them. The child-care expert Dr Penelope Leach, herself a mother, recognizes some of the dangers inherent in this situation:

Somehow the mother has to find ways of staying on the infant's side; of refusing to allow herself to feel against him; of nipping her own resentment in the bud and finding other ways of venting her stresses. Unfortunately our society's ideal is of the mother vho mothers sensitively and likes it. To admit that you cannot or do not enjoy this stage of mothering is to admit to a kind of failure . . . If welfare authorities, husbands and friends knew this, and could admire mothers for managing it, rather than taking it for granted as 'natural', that in itself would make the job seem a little easier.[1]

In fact the care of babies and young children is a highly skilled job and like other skills has to be learned. In more primitive and sociable societies it is learned by young girls watching older women breastfeeding and caring for the young. In our society, which considers breastfeeding in public as at best embarrassing and at worst disgusting, young girls have no opportunity to watch and learn the skills involved. We then show great concern that so many women are unable to breastfeed successfully and miss the irony of women failing to do something which is supposed to be instinctive.

The human female is not unique in this situation. Laboratory-raised monkeys who have been reared on their own have been found to be inefficient breastfeeders. Laboratory-raised monkeys are also inept at copulation, another form of supposedly 'instinctive' behaviour which has to be learned. Some human couples applying for adoption have been discovered to be childless because they simply did not know that penile penetration was necessary for conception.

There are no hormonal changes during the process of pregnancy and birth which equip a mother to know how to feed and care for her baby. Even love does not of itself teach us how to bring baby and breast together efficiently nor how to quiet a screaming baby or stimulate a quiet one. Women who come from large families have a built-in advantage over those who don't since they have watched and learned from their own mothers. The rest of us have to learn, slowly, painfully and often alone, how to cope with the conflicting practical and emotional demands of motherhood. One of these conflicts is explained by the sociologist Ann Oakley, in her book on housewives:

Children are directly antithetical to the demands of the housewife role: they are neither tidy nor clean in their 'natural' state . . . Being a 'good' mother does not call for the same qualities as being a 'good' housewife, and the pressure to be both at the same time may be an insupportable burden. Children may suffer because the goals of housework may become the goals of child care, and a dedication to keeping children clean and tidy may override an interest in their separate development as individuals.[2]

The houseworked child does credit to her mother since she is always neat, clean, polite and obedient. She never embarrasses her mother in public or disturbs the all-important adult world. Dorothy Edwards's sad portrait of Winnie in *My Naughty Little Sister* accurately captures such a child:

So my little sister said, 'Shall we have a race round the

lawn?' and Winnie said, 'Oh, no, it's *so* hot,' in a quiet good voice. And she didn't want to climb up the apple-trees in case she tore her frock, and she didn't want to sit in the grass in case there were ants, and she didn't want to shout over the front gate to the school children because it was rude, and all the time she just looked peepy, peepy at my little sister.

So then my little sister said, 'What would you like to do?' And the polite good Winnie said she would like to take a story-book indoors to read. So she took one of the story-books indoors and read on her own.[3]

When housework is lumped together with motherhood and when children create so much housework the mother is in a constant situation of conflict. It is usually assumed that the mother who is at home all day is lavishing time and attention on her child. She is in fact more likely to be washing, ironing, cleaning, dusting, polishing, preparing food or washing up. Those mothers who abandon the housework and con-centrate on stimulating their children are none too popular either: 'I feel that I'm got-at a lot of the time for not even doing what I'm doing very well because the place is a tip at certain times. That's a really frustrating thing.'

This lack of appreciation reflects the low status of both motherhood and housework. There was a time, before the last war, when married women were not allowed to work, when the birth of a first child brought enhanced status. Now that married women are used to the independent status of a job and a wage packet, this is no longer the case. However menial the job may be, at least it is recognized as work and carries some of the dignity of labour. Housework doesn't and being a mother means being a housewife: 'Once you have children people tend to think of you as less intelligent than when you didn't have children.' Domesticity is con-sidered trivial and boring and domestics soon become treated in the same way: 'I find that men always talk to me about the child. They always say "How's the little man" or something absolutely revolting and I say, "Oh, he's fine". I never really say anything else because I don't always want to talk about him and they never think that I can talk about anything else.

That really irritates me.'

This loss of status brought about by loss of income is in many ways similar to that of the unemployed man. There is the same demoralization, the same feeling that what money is received is not your own to spend, the same erosion of confidence in your own ability to hold down a job again, the same dropping out of previous activities. The difference is that the unemployed man has no other role to compensate for the loss of a job, whereas the housewife has a role which is stressful, exhausting and unappreciated: 'It's something to do with achievements. At the end of the day I often think what my husband has achieved to some extent, compared with me. There's no real achievement, I don't think.' Despite the very real moments of pleasure which can come from being with the baby and watching her grow, it can all seem endless. Time loses its sense of purpose because each day is like the last and will be like the next:

> And this tremendous stretch of time from your husband going off in the morning to coming in at night, perhaps at six. You've got too much to do but it's all the same. You read about these intellectual women who propped their Proust over the washing-up bowl and carried on with their reading, but they're in a great minority. Most of us are too damned tired to keep any sort of intellectual activity going.

The tiredness and continual activity needed to fit in housework with four-hour feeds leads easily to isolation. As one woman defined motherhood, 'Whatever you're invited to do, it's easier not to.' It's easier not to go out than to find a babysitter; it's easier not to travel because feeds are difficult to time; it's easier not to visit friends than to pack up everything that might be needed.

The world shrinks, inevitably and very rapidly, to four walls and a few streets. It is difficult to make new friends because it's not easy to get out of the house and there are few ready-made communities waiting to welcome the new mother. In her research into the conflicts of housebound mothers, *The Captive Wife*, published in 1966, Hannah Gavron discovered that none of the wives in her sample engaged in the kind of 'street life' traditionally associated with working-class urban life: 'This depends on a stable population, familiar with the area and its inhabitants, a street-level front door, reasonable safety from traffic, and perhaps most important of all a large number of home-based women, available during the day.'[4] She further comments that the working-class wives in her sample appeared to accept their role as mothers much more readily in theory but were in fact psychologically unprepared for the results. Their attitudes and expectations of motherhood seemed to come from the old patterns of extended family street life. In fact they suffered from a fair degree of isolation, reduced contacts with extended families due to the difficulties of travelling with children and experienced loneliness through the contrast between their present existence as mothers and their previous existence as working wives.

As people have moved away from their home towns in search of work, or have been rehoused in blocks of flats, so the street communities have dwindled. Life has always been physically very hard for working-class women but they have usually managed somehow to support each other. As one woman commented: 'The working classes had this community. There was never any question of you couldn't go to the pub with your old man for a drink because you hadn't a baby-sitter. You just shouted through the wall, "Will you listen for mine?" or you picked him up and dumped him in the cot with next door's. All that has now gone.'

There are few home-based women any more, most return to work as soon as they can. Traffic makes the streets dangerous for children. 'Keep the under-fives indoors' admonish the road safety adverts. Keep them at home where they are likely to have more accidents than anywhere else. Of course accidents in the home can always be blamed on the mother who has nowhere else for her child to play. The car driver who rules the streets doesn't need to worry about that.

Lack of safe playing space for children close to home is an additional stress for the housebound mother, especially if she has a new baby to cope with as well as a toddler. One study of the effects of housing on pre-school children and their mothers concluded that in both the groups living in high-rise and low-rise flats there were more mothers who complained of depression and loneliness and that in both groups there was significantly more dissatisfaction with their housing, especially the lack of playing space for children.[5]

In ordering our priorities, however, it is men first and women and children last. The men who sit on the planning and housing committees have more important things to consider than the needs of small children:

> All the feelings of discontent came to a head in the demonstrations which followed the child's accident. An ambitious toddler had climbed the three foot six balcony to have a peek at the world below, but leant too far out. The housing department were reluctant to rehouse his family, reluctant to set a precedent in humanity. It was only because we demonstrated and began to organize ourselves, that anything happened.[6]

Well, after all, you can't expect a busy housing department to concern themselves about toddlers falling off balconies or isolated and depressed mothers, can you? The housing department can only help to create the problems, it is the social services department that is responsible for sorting them out, or perhaps the police or the local psychiatric hospital.

There still are areas in Britain where the old working-class street communities continue to provide help and support for young mothers. In all too many areas, however, massive slum clearance programmes have replaced them with concrete wastelands where neighbourly contact is restricted to draughty corridors or badly maintained lifts; where there are few shops and poor bus services. None of these conditions create depression in themselves but they provide a fertile soil in which the seeds can grow.

As they say in the North, 'If you have nowt, you are nowt'; a good, blunt way of expressing the dominant values of our society. It is therefore not surprising that Professor Brown in his research into the social origins of depression discovered that working-class women are four times more likely to develop severe depression as a response to traumatic events than middle-class women. They are more likely to suffer from bad housing and severe financial difficulties and when disaster strikes in the form of a bereavement, separation or husband's unemployment, they have fewer resources to bolster their self-esteem.[7] If the working-class community cannot rally round to support its own, that mountain of sand will crush and suffocate.

Middle-class women have different problems. If poverty doesn't get you, affluence will. Margaret Dennis, who helped to found the Oxford Mothers' Group and is an experienced lay counsellor, told me:

It's an atmosphere in society now of self-sufficiency. You *ought* to be able to cope. I think it goes hand in hand with the general improvement in the standard of living. If you've got two cars outside the house and double glazing you *ought* to be able to cope with your emotional problems too. It's this *ought* thing. 'I've got a good husband, a comfortable home, wall-to-wall carpets, why am I like this? It's terrible, it's shameful, it's awful, I'll just opt out.' I say to girls on estates who are suicidal, 'How many women in the road are there with babies? Why don't you get together?' and they say, 'Well, I don't like to. She looks as if she's coping and I don't want to say I can't cope.' There's this ridiculous hang-up we've got about self-sufficiency, even towards husbands. They don't tell their husbands or their immediate family.

Middle-class women may have better housing, often with a garden for the child to play in. They have telephones to help ward off isolation (47 per cent of homes in Britain still don't have a telephone) and perhaps a car to help them travel farther afield. On the other hand they also have a better education which makes them feel keenly their decline in status to 'just a housewife' and they are likely to know very little about babies.

Hannah Gavron notes that 81 per cent of her middle-class sample had no previous experience of children or babies. The impact of the birth of the first child on the middle-class woman had been tremendous because it had changed them from being independent women into being traditional women. They all felt the need for a degree of independence and 92 per cent intended to return to work when the youngest child was at school.[8]

The middle-class woman is also confronted with the problem of isolation:

> In the old days you had help in the house, help with the housework if you were middle class. The upper classes didn't deal with children at all, they just handed them over. The middle classes are now left with an enormous void. You haven't got mother and family because you've probably moved away. Or you've been educated to think, 'I've grown up now, I've left home, and this is my life, I'm not going to turn to my mother and say "Please help".' You can't afford even someone to come in and help you in the mornings with the housework, and that would be another woman, an older woman with experience who could look at the nappy rash and say, 'Oh, yes, all mine had that, it's nothing.' You haven't got that. You're left, you're on your own.

The new private housing estate where everyone is busy keeping up standards is often more competitive than supportive. Margaret Dennis comments: 'I don't get so many girls with depression on council estates as I get on private estates, you know, little separated detached boxes with a tiny little street; straining to pay the mortgage, straining to keep up.' The pleasant, leafy suburb breeds many a smiling depression. As one mother described it: 'You had to go about with that big smile on your face and people saying, "Aren't you *lucky* to have such a dear little baby," and you feel utter despair.'

Despite the differences in both material circumstances and attitudes between working-class and middle-class women, there is much which they have in common. Both groups suffer from the problems of isolation, both have to cope with the conflicts of housework and child care, both share the low status of housewives and both are financially dependent on either husbands or the state. Hannah Gavron notes that both her samples were aware of the conflict over their roles as *mother* and *worker* though neither saw any great conflict between their roles as *wife* and *worker*.[9]

The mother-at-home risks loneliness, boredom and feelings of fragmentation and demoralization:

> When the baby was about five months old, I began to feel as if he was a kind of monster, almost swallowing me up in his demands. I felt as if 'I' was disappearing and that I would never be a person in my own right again, even though I knew the baby needed me to make advances and responses to him so that he could develop.

This feeling of being nothing, of losing yourself, can be the start of a depression. Self-esteem is not possible if there is no sense of self. On the other hand the working mother has to cope with a constant, nagging guilt. In addition she has the double workload of house, child and job. Despite this, Professor Brown identifies employment as offering some protection against the onset of depression in women, possibly by increasing their sense of self-esteem.

Another study of mental distress in mothers of pre-school children, conducted by Peter Moss and Ian Plewis of the Thomas Coram Institute, does not confirm this protective relationship. They did, however, find a significant relationship between distress in mothers and a desire to start work now, expressed by women at home full-time.[10] This finding confirms that of yet another study which discovered that mothers with pre-school children who felt a duty to stay at home but didn't enjoy it and wanted to work were four times as likely to have been given sedatives and tranquillizers in the previous year as those who felt no such conflict.[11]

Moss and Plewis comment that if further studies confirm a causal relationship between mental health and wanting to go to work, this has serious implications for the next five years or so. In this period it seems likely that labour market demand for women with children will be, at best, static and, at worst, decreasing, while the numbers of mothers wanting to work will rise. As a consequence there will be an increase in the numbers of mothers experiencing conflict between home ties and an unfulfilled desire to work.[12]

It is not, perhaps, so easy to use married women as a cheap pool of reserve labour as some might have supposed. The expectations of women have changed and the realities of motherhood fail to match up to its romantic image.

Like the pieces of a Chinese puzzle, there fits within the mother-worker conflict yet another conflict which is neatly pinned down by the psychologist Ann Dally: 'The particular conflict of women in the modern world is that good mothering tends to prevent that personal development and liberation without which it is impossible to be a good mother.'[13] What this means is that mothers who stay at home in order to look after their children find it difficult to develop as people, and mothers who are unable to develop as people cannot achieve the distance from their children which is necessary for eventual separation. She adds: 'Motherhood is part of women's destiny but it is only a part. Few women find total fulfilment in it for more than short periods of time. If they do, then . . . they are likely to be inadequate not only as people but also as mothers, and emotionally dependent on their children.'[14]

Obviously many women do manage to resolve this conflict, but it is by no means easy:

When I'm working I have the feeling that it would be nice just to be a placid Mum at home with plenty of time and when I'm at home, obviously, I feel absolutely the reverse. When I started the job I'm in at the moment, I was only working three days a week and people used to say, 'Isn't that marvellous, you've absolutely got the best of both worlds,' whereas in fact, at that stage I felt frustrated because a three-day working week passes exceedingly quickly and you always have the feeling that you've never got anything done. So then I swopped to working four days a week and had the reverse feeling that I never had any time at home. I'm quite happy to live with this level of frustration because I don't think there's anything one can do about it.

In traditional societies where there is little social change the demands made of mothers are relatively simple. When the son of a farmer becomes a farmer and his daughter marries a farmer, then the job of the mother is simply to rear children according to traditional values with practical agricultural skills. She does not need to separate herself from them since they will remain within the community as part of the extended family. It is a static and limiting situation but at least it is secure.

In a society where there is rapid social change and a philosophy of equality of opportunity, the demands made of mothers are very much greater. Children must develop as mature, flexible, independent individuals and not be held back by a possessive or domineering mother.

The changing views of child-care experts probably have more to do with the changing values of society than the scientific study of child development. Truby King, writing at the turn of the century, reflected the ideals of his time: 'If we lack noble mothers we lack the first element of racial success and national greatness.'[15] And the methods he exhorted these noble mothers to use were routine, regularity and absolute control, starting from birth. He stipulated clock-like regularity of feeding, regularity of exercise, bathing, sleeping and action of the bowels. He castigated the 'can't-be-so-cruel' mother:

> The can't-be-so-cruel mother, whose baby cries half the night and frets all day on account of the mother's failure to fulfil one of the first maternal duties, should not blame Providence or heredity because her progeny has turned out a 'simply-won't' in infancy, and will become a selfish 'simply-can't' in later childhood and adolescence. Power to obey the 'Ten Commandments', or to conform to the temporal laws and usage of society, is not to be expected of 'spoiled' babies when they reach adult life.[16]

Today the ideals of racial success and national greatness would not find too many supporters. We live in a different world with different values, and ideas about child rearing have changed. We are now encouraged to demand-feed babies, potty-train them later and respond to them as individuals. Whether all this advice makes much difference is open to question. As Ann Dally points out: 'What a mother is is much more important than what she does. This fact is usually omitted in books and articles on child care.'[17] Like the song says, it's not what you do, it's the way that you do it, and a frustrated, unhappy mother won't do any of it with much enjoyment.

In their study, Moss and Plewis defined 'moderate distress' by such things as taking a course of 'psychiatric' drugs; feeling life was not worth living; or having appetite, sleep and one other physical function affected for more than a week. 'Severe distress' they defined by such things as admission to mental hospital; a suicide attempt; a strongly expressed inability to cope with day-to-day life; or feelings of depersonalization. Fifty-two per cent of mothers had suffered from moderate or severe distress in the twelve months prior to interview and 37 per cent for the four weeks immediately preceding the interview. Forty-nine per cent of the women with moderate distress and 30 per cent of the women with severe distress had not sought help.[18]

The women in this study were women with children under five and they were asked about their emotional state only in the previous twelve months. Since there is no indication when their distress started it is not possible to say whether it can be called postnatal depression. Since 43 per cent of Pitt's depressed mothers had not improved after a year[19] it is not unreasonable to assume that a proportion of these distressed women were suffering from postnatal depression. In practice the distinction is not very important since all depressed mothers need care. It would nonetheless be interesting to know at what point after birth most of these women started to become distressed and for how long the mood persisted. However, considering the lack of medical research there has been into postnatal depression, it is encouraging to find community studies appearing to fill the gap.

If a man who had just won the Marathon was then allowed only three hours' sleep at a stretch for the next six weeks whilst being expected to perform during the day a series of boring, repetitive tasks in isolation and was constantly told throughout that he ought to be happy because he'd just won the Marathon, we might imagine some fiendish political regime was trying to break him. Yet women, after the immense physical effort of birth, face precisely these conditions and are expected to cope. Margaret Dennis feels strongly about this:

> I think that the primary cause which is underestimated, I would say 100 per cent by male doctors, is fatigue, just sheer physical exhaustion. Some of them have the imagination to be able to realize in their heads at least what it's like to be on the go all day with a very demanding two-year-old, and it really is a killing age to have *all* day, and then a baby who gets you up at regular intervals throughout the night. Some of them can imagine what that is like but a lot of them can't. It's like medieval torture isn't it? After all, it is used. They used it in Northern Ireland, they use it in countries all over the world. They wake you up every time you go to sleep and you'll do and say anything. It's better sometimes, I used to feel, not to go to bed at all because when you've just gone into that first deep, deep sleep, to be dragged out of it is to feel murderous.

Truby King absolutely forbade night-feeding. He claimed that it spoiled the baby and undermined the mother's health. He was probably correct in the latter, if not the former. It is obviously cruel to starve a newborn baby and yet it is essential for new mothers to recover from labour.

'I know this sounds a very trivial point but I'm convinced that all new mothers need just a night or two of absolutely guaranteed, undisturbed sleep to recover from labour and to set them up for the rigours which lie ahead,' one woman wrote to me, and her feelings would be echoed by many. There are, however, a substantial number of women who object to their babies being removed from them at any time whilst they are in hospital. The advantages of a rooming-in policy which keeps babies with their mothers all the time in the ward are that it enables mothers to get to know their babies and feel in control of feeds and routine. The disadvantage is that it leads to broken nights with babies waking to be fed at different intervals. At Charing Cross Hospital Dr Hugh Jolly, the consultant paediatrician, encourages mothers to keep their babies in bed with them, using baby slings. He claims that this reduces the crying, which it probably does if all mothers breastfeed. Hospital beds are high and narrow and hardly conducive to intimacy but since animal mothers manage to rest and suckle at the same time there is no reason why human mothers shouldn't be able to do so. If a choice has to be made, however, between twenty-four-hour contact with the baby and a good night's sleep, there is no question in my mind that sleep is the first essential for the new mother.

The tiredness got worse. Our very marriage was becoming a battleground. It was awful. I had made friends with a girl I met at relaxation classes and we swopped notes. She was so depressed she had been put on anti-depressant drugs. But was she depressed? *No.* Both of us were so dog tired the world was a mountain. Nine months later and both happy again, enjoying our babies and good marriages again, we agreed – it was the tiredness. If we could have slept the day after delivery, if we could have had more rest in the hospital – if, if, if. Many friends have said the same – you don't realize you're depressed, you just feel so tired.

There is very little opportunity for rest in hospital after having a baby. A woman who goes into labour say on Monday afternoon and delivers her baby in the early hours of Tuesday morning may find herself in the postnatal ward just as the hospital day is starting and be unable to sleep until the Tuesday evening. Her body will not only have been through the enormous effort of giving birth, it will also have been deprived of sleep for thirty-six hours. Sleep which is lost at this time is unlikely to be made up later:

I had a long labour, thirteen hours, and I was very tired afterwards. I never really got over the tiredness. Also, when he was born he was only 5 lb. 3½ oz. so it was difficult to feed him. I was feeding him myself and I had to be on three-hourly feeds. It used to take me two hours to feed him. You know I was absolutely worn out. Then he had jaundice, he had colic, he had thrush. He had the lot in that first three months and we didn't get any sleep for three months because he just screamed night and day.

Even without the additional problems of a sickly small baby to cope with, feeding alone can keep you up half the night: 'I also felt very tired because the baby didn't sleep through the night until she was six weeks old. She took 1½ hours each feed, usually two a.m. and six a.m. and I felt that one feed was only over when another was due.' Exhaustion can lead inevitably to isolation since it becomes impossible, without energy, to get out anywhere. Lack of sleep also undermines physical resistance and disturbs the balance of the mind. The problem is that lethargy and tiredness are in themselves symptoms of depression.

The tiredness of depression is like energy swallowed. It goes underground, somewhere out of reach. One depressed person described it as two horses at war in the mind. The conflict is buried, forgotten and so, like a kind of spiritual cramp, our whole being is locked in pain, exhausted and incapable of doing anything to help itself. The trolls have stolen our gold and left us without the means to look for it. We move through endless circles in the mind; like walking on the moors in the fog, we exhaust ourselves and return, unnourished, to the starting point again.

It is not easy to define the point at which physical fatigue due to weeks of broken nights and daily housework turns into the lethargy of depression, though it is easy to see how it puts women at risk. There are many pieces to that stained glass window and exhaustion is only one of them; for some women, perhaps the largest one. Certainly it is something which should be avoidable in the 1970s. There are still working women today who carry far too heavy a workload during pregnancy and have no one to help in the home when they leave hospital. We must not forget the terrible lessons of our grandmothers' and great grandmothers' lives:

The first part of my life I spent in a screw factory from six in the morning till five at night; and after tea used to do my washing and cleaning. I only left two weeks and three weeks before my first children were born. After that I took in lodgers and washing, and always worked up till an hour or so before baby was born. The results are that three of my girls suffer with their insides. None are able to have a baby. One dear boy was born ruptured on account of my previous hard work . . . I could never afford a nurse, and so was a day or two after my confinements obliged to sit up and wash and dress the others.

My husband's wages varied owing to either hot weather or some of the other men not working . . . I had three little ones in two years and five months, and he was out of work two years, and during that time I took in washing and sewing and have not been near a bed for night after night. I was either at my sewing machine or ironing after the little ones had gone to bed. After being confined five days I have had to do all for my little ones. I worked sometimes up till a few moments before they were born. I do hope I have not done wrong in relating so much of my past, and that it may be of some use in the furthering of our scheme.[20]

11. 'A Woman's Place is in the Wrong'*

According to Greek legend, the hero, Theseus, in his travels as a young man, met and killed a robber named Procrustes. Procrustes enticed travellers to his home where he made them lie upon a bed. If they were too tall for the bed, he lopped off their limbs; and if too short, he stretched their limbs until they were long enough.

The feminine and maternal role is a Procrustean bed; we cannot, as individuals, fit it and we suffer in one way or another when we don't. Despite the very high rates of depression evident in mothers, the physical constraints, the ideas and ideals which form the bed they are fitted on, which, indeed, support the institutions of marriage and the family, continue.

The conditioned reflex of history is to blame women for not fitting the bed and thus cut them down to size. In this way mothers have been blamed not only for their own suffering but for most of the evil, foolishness, insanity and crime infecting human society: 'If women in general were rendered more fit for maternity . . . the main supply of population for our asylums, hospitals, benevolent institutions, gaols and slums would be cut off at source.'[1] It is an old prejudice and one which has no evidence to support it. It inflicts endless guilt and misery on mothers struggling to do the best they can in difficult circumstances and it totally ignores the individual needs and differences of women.

According to Leviticus, once a year the Jewish high priest symbolically laid the sins of the people upon a goat which was allowed to escape into the wilderness. This was the scapegoat which has come to mean the person who carries the blame due to others. Scapegoats are usually groups or individuals who have the least power in society and can therefore be safely blamed without threat of reprisal. Women are

* Attributed to W. C. Fields.

easy scapegoats. Unlike the ethnic minorities who can be seen as groups with definite identities, women are rarely viewed as a group because they are split up, attached to individual men, hidden in the home.

The persecution of racial minorities as scapegoats has been frequent and hideous. Racism and anti-semitism run through history and can be clearly seen. The persecution of women, apart from the witch hunts of the Middle Ages and the brutal attacks on suffragettes, including forced feeding, has gener- ally been more hidden. As problems occur, women are picked off individually. Things have gone wrong because there is something wrong with us. We are to blame for not being better mothers, better wives, better in bed, less anxious, less tired. And when others blame us so much is it really any wonder that we blame ourselves?

Because guilt and self-reproach are such an inevitable and harmful part of depression, I think it is important to look in detail at both the Procrustean methods of treating mothers and the ways in which women generally are used as scapegoats.

We are supposed to think of motherhood in terms of serene and lovely madonnas, the laughing young women of the corn-flake advertisements, the sensitive, patient, eternally loving mothers of the child-care books, always married, always well housed. We are supposed to think of motherhood as something which all women are equally suited to and which all women want to do. We are not supposed to think of the women who risk their health at back-street abortionists; of the women driven to abandon their babies in lifts, parks or outside hospitals; of the pregnant teenage girl kicked out by her family. We are not supposed to think of motherhood in terms of hopelessness, depression, violence.

The unmarried mother, the teenage mother, the depressed mother, the 'battering' mother, the 'rejecting' mother: all are considered failures, deviant, abnormal, 'problems'; and in them all are fragments of ourselves. The ideal mother, like the ideal baby or the ideal labour, simply doesn't exist. Women who find great satisfaction in caring for their babies and toddlers need to resist a temptation to feel smug for who knows, they may yet be accused of smothering their adoles-cent children. We should always be aware of mothers with problems but beware of calling them 'problem mothers'.

In her book *Of Woman Born*, the American poet Adrienne Rich carefully defines the violence done to women by the institution of motherhood as distinct from the richness and depth of the experience of motherhood. Taking the case of a thirty-eight-year-old Chicago mother with eight children who killed her two youngest with a butcher's knife, she describes with passionate clarity the dark forces at the heart of motherhood, the suffering of the scapegoat:

> She loved, she tried to love, she screamed and was not heard, because there was nothing and no one in her surroundings who saw her plight as unnatural, as anything but the 'homemaker's' usual service to the home. She became a scapegoat, the one around whom the darkness of maternity is allowed to swirl – the invisible violence of the institution of motherhood, the guilt, the powerless responsibility for human lives, the judgments and condemnations, the fear of her own power, the guilt, the guilt, the guilt. So much of this heart of darkness is an undramatic, undramatized suffering: the woman who serves her family their food but cannot sit down with them, the woman who cannot get out of bed in the morning, the woman polishing the same place on the table over and over, reading labels in the supermarket as if they were in a foreign language, looking into a drawer where there is a butcher knife. The scapegoat is also an escape-valve: through her the passions and the blind raging waters of a suppressed knowledge are permitted to churn their way so that they need not emerge in less extreme situations as lucid rebellion. Reading of the 'bad' mother's desperate response to an invisible assault on her being, 'good' mothers resolve to become better, more patient and long-suffering, to cling more tightly to what passes for sanity. The scapegoat is different from the martyr; she cannot teach resistance or revolt. She represents a terrible temptation: to suffer uniquely, to assume that I, the individual woman, am the 'problem'.[2]

The prime purpose of this book is to try and ensure that

the suffering of depressed mothers is not solitary and is not seen to be unique. Whilst there is no shortage of experts willing to tell mothers what they should feel, there is also, fortunately, no shortage of mothers who know that most of it is idealized wishful thinking. The taboos of family loyalty, which have long prevented women from telling each other how they felt about their marriages and children, are slowly disappearing. There is an increased awareness amongst women of the kind of problems they share and an increased willingness to talk about them: 'You didn't talk about things like that at home in those days. I felt I was the only person in the world depressed. I've spoken to lots of people since . . . now everybody seems to be on tranquillizers or anti-depressants but nobody seemed to be then.' The more that women talk about and share their problems, the more aware they become of the kind of stresses they share. It is this shared knowledge which can give us the courage to break out of traditional formulas and solutions. It is this shared knowledge and support which can enable us to resist becoming scapegoats.

Since Eve first tempted Adam, women have been seen as dangerous temptresses leading men down the primrose path to hell. In order to control and rule over such fearful creatures men have been given tacit permission to beat the living day-lights out of them. Of all the violent crimes committed, it is most often those of men against women which are judged to have been 'provoked' by the victim. A young man mugged and beaten up after a football match is not told by the judge that it's his own fault for going to the match wearing the 'wrong' scarf and he only got what he deserved. Yet this is how rape victims are usually treated. The sympathies of our great, im-partial British legal system are tacitly on the side of the male assaulter in most cases of rape and marital violence.

Any woman of any age at any time can be the victim of a rape attack and in court, if she has the courage to prosecute, she will risk being accused of being a prostitute. In July 1977, summing up in a rape case where a fifteen-year-old girl was dragged from a bus stop by four boys and raped in the woods under threat of violent attack, the judge stated that parents

who allowed their young daughters to roam the streets of
South London like 'little harlots' carried most of the blame
for what happened to them.[3] The parents of the boys involved in this vicious attack were not blamed for allowing
their sons to roam the streets like wild animals. It should be
a matter of the gravest concern that any judge tacitly con-
dones brutality and violence against women in this way.

In cases of marital violence women are also held to blame
for 'provoking' attacks. In one case of vicious murder the
defence lawyer's comments showed the unthinking trivializa-
tion of violence in marriage. The wife, he said, had taunted
her husband and 'the pity of the matter is that the taunting
came when the hammer was in his hand. Otherwise it might
have been just one of those *trivial* incidents one hears about
in the divorce courts where the husband is *provoked* and *only
hits* his wife.'[4] (My italics.)

The lack of concern shown by the law and men in general
on both the issues of rape and wife beating give the lie to the
chivalrous idea of men protecting women. The bitter history
of the sex war shows that male protection is a racket. Thou
shalt not rape is not one of the Ten Commandments.[5] A man
may protect the woman he regards as his personal property
but only if she does as she is told and is always sexually
available. If she fails to conform she has only herself to blame
for the often violent consequences.

To atone for the sins of Eve, the temptress, women have
been made to tread the narrow path to salvation through
marriage and motherhood. Church and state joined together
to outcast the unmarried mother and her bastard child, leaving them destitute. Strict anti-abortion laws and the lack of
effective contraception led to desperate measures. The com-
monest crime in Western Europe from the Middle Ages
through to the end of the eighteenth century was the truly
tragic one of mothers killing their babies. Forced to bear
children which they could not rear, women in all lands
throughout the ages have been driven to destroy the new lives
they have borne.

Unmarried mothers still suffer from great social and economic pressures and are usually blamed for their own con-

dition. They 'get themselves pregnant' and the pregnancy is seen as a punishment. The punishment is, in fact, a baby and a baby at risk. The perinatal mortality rates show that twenty illegitimate babies die per 1000 births as compared to fourteen legitimate babies per 1000. There is also a high risk of prematurity and handicap in the babies of unsupported mothers. Margaret Bramall, ex-Director of the National Council for One-Parent Families, believes there are four main reasons for this situation: poverty; poor nutrition, frequently brought about by poverty; the fact that many young and unsupported mothers do not qualify for the maternity grant (poverty); and failure to seek adequate antenatal care usually because guilt prevents the unmarried mother from accepting the pregnancy and because antenatal services are unsympathetic and do nothing to encourage unsupported mothers to attend regularly.[6]

In terms of depression, 'non-married' mothers are also a very vulnerable group. Moss and Plewis discovered in their research into mental distress in mothers of pre-school children that 72 per cent of 'non-married' mothers either had or had been through a moderate or severe distress problem as compared with 46 per cent of 'married' mothers.[7]

Thus women continue to bear the major responsibility for sexual activity and its consequences. They are to blame for provoking desire in men and by consenting to sexual intercourse are held responsible for its consequences. This tacitly encourages sexual irresponsibility in men.

In addition women are generally blamed not only for their own frigidity but also for male impotence. Attitudes to our female sexuality, like our hemlines, have risen and fallen but always we have been to blame for not conforming sexually to what men believe is right and proper. In the Victorian era doctors believed that 'good' women didn't experience any sexual desire: 'As a general rule, a modest woman seldom desires any sexual gratification for herself. She submits to her husband's embraces, but principally to gratify him; and, were it not for the desire of maternity, would far rather be relieved from his attentions.'[8] This view of female sexuality was widely held in Victorian times and was, of course, transmitted from

mother to daughter. For the most part it was a silent communication which made it the more powerful. What cannot be
spoken of must be dangerous and wicked. Unbeknown to the
daughters of Victorian mothers, however, Sigmund Freud had
appeared on the scene.

The 'modest' woman who would rather be relieved of
her husband's advances was fast turning into that monster of
Freudian mythology, the frigid woman: 'Frigidity in sexual
intercourse occurs only in women whose relationships with
men are, in general, characterized by fear, hate, envy and
rejection; in short, in women who cannot love. Moreover,
their incapacity to love, although most manifest in their relationships with men, extends to all their human contacts . . .'[9]
This evil stereotype of the castrating, devouring, loveless
woman stalks the pages of psychoanalytic writing like the
demonic Lilith of Hebrew myth.[10] Despite the findings of the
Kinsey Report in 1953 that orgasm without stimulation is a
physical impossibility for nearly all women, female psychology
continues to be blamed.

Common sense and common experience might suggest that
lack of sex education, feelings about sex being dirty or simply
poor stimulation and technique on the part of lovers might
go a long way to explaining frigidity. Indeed the same vicious
trio might go a long way to explaining impotence in men as
well. Despite this, male impotence is also blamed in one way
or another on women:

> The male is a fragile creature sexually. If women have been
> forced by the advent of the permissive society to feel
> prudish if they say no, the poor man has not only to 'get it
> up' and provide multiple orgasms on demand – but with
> all this fake, rattle and roll around cannot even be sure
> he's giving any pleasure. No wonder the doctors' waiting-
> rooms are full of cases of impotence.[11]

So writes Jilly Cooper in a review of *The Hite Report*, an
American study of sexuality in 3000 women which revealed
that only 30 per cent reported having regular orgasms from
intercourse.[12] This is really just another version of the old 'castrating woman' threat usually hurled at feminists and free-

thinking women. It presupposes that men are incapable of handling strong, independent women without wilting on the spot and it grossly over-simplifies the problem of impotence.

More specifically, some doctors have blamed impotence on lack of attractiveness in wives. One such doctor claims to take determined and somewhat drastic action: 'I treat the women and not the virtually impotent man. Sometimes a simple consultation is enough to eliminate sexual difficulties, such as sending the wife to the dentist, coiffeur, or tailor, etc. Sometimes hormonal treatment is necessary (e.g. in obesity) or surgical (e.g. narrow or large vagina).'[13] It is interesting how often doctors are attracted by the idea of using surgery on female genitals. It is to be hoped in this case that the wife so conveniently tailored to suit her husband doesn't decide to leave him for a man of different proportions.

Since priests, philosophers and doctors have never hesitated to tell women exactly what they should feel without ever bothering to consult them, it is not surprising to find that women are blamed for not experiencing their lives in the way they should.

Feeling is one of the few totally spontaneous activities. It cannot be ordered or controlled by act of will though the expressions of it can. This means that women fake orgasm, fake love, fake obedience whilst repressing feelings of anger, self-loathing and despair. Writing of the myth and cult of the Virgin Mary, Marina Warner comments that: '... the types of virtues decreed feminine degenerate easily: obedience becomes docility; gentleness, irresolution; humility, cringing; forbearance, long-suffering.'[14] The attempt to mould women into noble and virtuous creatures according to an imposed pattern and without understanding the real nature of their experience simply produces a mockery of the ideal.

The utter pointlessness of telling women what they can and should feel about sex and motherhood has not yet entered the blinkered view of many psychologists. Instead they busily label and categorize the thousand conflicting realities of women's lives under headings of 'refusal of femininity' or 'failure to adjust to the maternal and feminine role'. The afflictions which are supposed to assail women who fail to fit this Procrustean bed are so numerous and include such common ailments as period pains, premenstrual tension, nausea in pregnancy, cystitis and, of course, postnatal depression, that we can rest assured that according to these definitions almost all of us are failing in one way or another to be feminine and/ or maternal.

It seems quite clear that when doctors don't actually know the cause of a particular condition, prejudice can encourage them to blame the woman herself for causing it. In their book *Hard Labour,* the doctors Jean and John Lennane describe the way in which this unconscious prejudice works by a process which they call 'reverse thinking'. Reverse thinking sees the reaction to an ailment as its cause. Thus fear of menstruation is said to 'cause' painful periods rather than the fear being seen as a direct result of the experience of the pain. One of the classic examples of this reverse thinking which they quote comes from the days when thousands of women died after childbirth as a result of puerperal fever. We know now that puerperal fever was caused by bacteria and spread by doctors examining women without modern antiseptic precautions. It was understandably a much-feared risk of childbirth and it was claimed that this fear, in itself, caused the fever:

> Few women die in labour, though many lose their lives after it; which may be thus accounted for. A woman after delivery, finding herself weak and exhausted, immediately apprehends she is in danger; but this fear seldom fails to obstruct the necessary evacuations, upon which her recovery depends. Thus the sex fall a sacrifice to their own imaginations, when there would be no danger, did they apprehend none.[15]

The danger of this kind of approach to illness in women is that it can lead to real organic illness being ignored or treated with tranquillizers. In 1972 it was estimated that 20 per cent of the American adult female population was given tranquillizers for the same diseases that men were given medicine for.[16] Examples are migraine, headache, abdominal pains and fatigue. One American medical textbook called *Obstetrics and Gynae-*

cology goes so far as to tell students that 'post-menopausal women who have been separated from significant men in their lives . . . may have vaginal bleeding', which is especially dangerous since in this age-group vaginal bleeding is one of the signs of uterine cancer.[17]

Since British women are treated by general practitioners rather than having to go to specialists as most American women do, we probably manage to escape some of the worst excesses of the gynaecologist. It also seems that by dint of national temperament, the National Health Service or poverty, or all three, we have managed to be less thoroughly soaked in popularized Freudian ideas than the Americans. I find it difficult to imagine a book like Erica Jong's *Fear of Flying*, which is saturated in psychoanalytic thought, being written by a British novelist. Nonetheless, even a practical, down-to-earth family doctor can be blinded by prejudice against women and dismiss their problems as self-inflicted. This is serious enough when a woman's health is at stake, but becomes increasingly serious when a child's health is also involved.

One woman recently told me about her child who had been continuously sick as a baby and had later developed severe stomach pains. The mother had brought her to the doctor and the hospital repeatedly and had been told the trouble was 'psychological'. Because the child was in pain the mother persisted, however, and finally when she was five years old a new doctor diagnosed a double hernia, 'probably present from birth', and the child was admitted to hospital for surgery. Another case which was brought to my notice was that of a mother who was treated with tranquillizers because she believed her baby was deaf. Nearly two years later when the little girl failed to talk it was discovered that she was indeed partially deaf. There is no way, in the absence of medical proof, that a mother can show that her anxieties are genuine. Yet a mother's anxiety is the only protection a child has. Labelling women as 'neurotic' when they are simply worried about a sick child is indefensible. It trivializes the genuine love and concern of the mother. Whenever the refrain 'it's all your fault!' is used it is usually a cover for 'I don't know'.

Some doctors seem to find it intolerable to have to admit that medical science cannot provide the answer to all problems.

The study of psychosomatic medicine is the study of the way the mind (*psyche*) affects the body (*soma*) and the body the mind. We tend to hear more about 'nervous headaches' and 'nervous stomachs' than we do about an attack of 'flu producing feelings of depression or even depression resulting from reaction to hormones in the contraceptive pill, but nonetheless psychosomatic reactions do work both ways round. One psychiatrist I talked to said that he always conducted a thorough gynaecological examination of all women who came to him suffering from postnatal depression, which seemed to me eminently sensible.

There are many theories about psychosomatic illness, especially in relation to women, but remarkably little real evidence. This can lead to the curious situation of some 'body' doctors treating physical symptoms as though they were mentally caused whilst most 'mind' doctors treat mental disorders as though they were a physical illness. Certainly, as far as the theories about psychosomatic illness are concerned, researchers frequently talk in terms of 'failure to adjust to the maternal and feminine role' as the chief cause of conflict. It takes an exceptionally perceptive doctor to see that 'success in adjusting to the maternal and feminine role' is a more likely cause. One GP, writing of a patient suffering from migraine and nausea comments:

> Doris has spent her life anticipating and responding to other people's demands and feelings but discounting and swallowing her own. Of course such a pattern of passivity is strongly reinforced by others who would probably describe her as 'a conscientious worker', 'such a *nice* woman', or 'a wonderful wife to John'. But the price for such outer charm and compliance is her inner rage and rebellion and even that she will only express by her incapacity and unconscious body language.[18]

There is no real proof that his diagnosis is correct, though I suspect it is closer to the truth than most. If Doris's problem is psychosomatic, at least he sees in her the suffering of a woman who has cut off a part of herself in order to try and fit the Procrustean bed of 'femininity' defined as self-sacrifice, compliance, submission and passivity.

There is further evidence, in Dana Breen's research into well-adjusted mothers, that success in adjusting to conventionally defined femininity can lead to problems. She used the Franck drawing test to try and discover the meaning of pregnancy and the birth of a first child for a woman's sense of femininity. This test consists of a number of incomplete drawings which a person completes as she likes. Drawings which are completed to expand outwards or to represent active movement are scored as male and drawings which are completed in an enclosed way or which represent passive containers such as vases are scored as female. This test claims to be culture-free and to relate to body image, which is why she chose to use it. She discovered, however, that it was the ill-adjusted women who had the highest femininity scores using this test and the well-adjusted women who had the highest masculinity scores. She comments that this put in doubt not so much the test itself as the interpretation Kate Franck put on its power to discriminate between the sexes:

> It seems legitimate to question this self image of passivity as representing feminine nature, since it turns out to be maladaptive to childbearing, the most feminine activity. Adjustment to pregnancy and the birth of a child is more likely to be linked to a sense of being in control, of being the active partner, being creative, being a giver rather than to a sense of being passive, someone who is held, contained, given to.[19]

She further found that the women with low 'femininity' scores felt positively that the baby was really theirs whilst the reverse was true of the women with high 'femininity' scores, something which she feels is related to the way women experienced giving birth.

It is possible that, given time, research into psychosomatic illness will be conducted with a different set of values; that definitions of femininity and the role which women are being expected to adapt to will be more critically examined than they are at present.

The threat of being found neurotic hangs over all mothers, but especially if they are educated and middle-class. Whilst biological myth-making permits mothers to be aggressive in defence of their young ('it seems to be true that aggression in the female is only fully aroused in response to threat, especially if the young are involved,' writes Anthony Storr in *Human Aggression*[20]), such aggression is not, somehow, supposed to apply to the doctor who won't allow her to hold her baby or the hospital who won't allow her to stay with her sick child. Nor, incidentally, is such aggression supposed to apply to local education authorities who fail to supply adequate schools or planners who fail to supply safe road crossings, or indeed to any male authority which puts the safety and happiness of children somewhere at the bottom of its list of priorities. In these situations female aggression is quite definitely 'neurotic'.

Such a liberal use of the clinical term 'neurotic' to smear all women who fail to be continuously serene and compliant has rendered the word virtually meaningless. We no longer see the genuine suffering of the truly neurotic woman as anything to be concerned about. It takes an experienced and humane psychiatrist like Jack Dominian to remind us of our callousness:

> People with a neurotic disposition are as talented, gifted, intelligent as the rest of the population, if not more so. They happen as a group to have a greater tendency towards the experiences and manifestations of certain characteristics such as anxiety, mood swings, low threshold to pain and a sensitivity to stress which they experience more easily and to a greater degree than others. To dismiss their suffering or distress as fake, or to pass adverse opinions on their behaviour is an unwarranted moral judgment without factual foundation.[21]

Neurotic or not, we are led to believe that if we raise our children with continuous love and patience, we can change the face of human society. This may be true, but since no one seriously expects us to succeed, the lofty ideals of motherhood are in fact just a scourge to beat us with and keep us in our places. Imagine then the consternation of the professionals when one amazing mother actually succeeds!

In the early 1970s a television producer, Michael Deakin, in the course of doing research for a documentary programme, came to a dilapidated cottage in deepest Wales. He found there four extraordinary children. Christian, aged twelve, already had A-levels in mathematics and science. Adam, aged nine, had won a national piano-playing contest open to children aged up to eighteen. Ruth, aged seven, painted brilliant pictures and Paul, aged five, wrote out his sums in Fortran, a computer language. The amazing intellectual development of these children came as a result of the deliberate decision of their mother, Maria, supported by her husband, to embark on the task of rearing happy, non-violent people.

In his book *The Children on the Hill*, Michael Deakin explains how this remarkable mother created in her remote cottage a prepared environment where she could catch each sign of a new development in her children and encourage it. In order to do this she had to live in isolation from other adults and survive on only four or five hours' sleep a night. The children were never smacked or spoken to in anger; they did not know what the word 'naughty' meant. When a baby threw its rattle out of the cot, she would pick it up, wash it, and return it for the baby to throw out again. This was repeated a hundred or more times until the baby had learned what he or she needed to learn. Such a formidable commitment produced great strain:

It is true that these difficulties have from time to time threatened to overwhelm her and that she has suffered periods of psychological disruption and acute mental and physical exhaustion. But a lesser woman would never have embarked on a scheme whose basic precepts involved total isolation and total self-sacrifice, and it is hard to imagine anybody else with the strength, albeit engendered by the unswerving calm and commitment of her husband, to carry such burdens for upwards of ten years.

But she did it, and did it in the belief that she could eradicate the darker sides of human behaviour; in the belief that what we mostly accept as being 'natural' could be proved to be the result of avoidable strains during early development. Since the children are not yet grown we cannot know if her belief was correct, but she certainly achieved what all mothers have been exhorted to achieve. And yet, alas, even she is open to condemnation for not failing:

> Up to the present she has been successful – the children are as strikingly *different* as their upbringing has been; and different in quality as well as in educational excellence. Professional outsiders tend to take the view that this very difference is in itself dangerous for the children; that far from representing the vanguard of a new type of individual, as their mother hopes, they are bound to become social casualties. The argument is simple – they are so qualitatively apart, that when the time comes not only to leave their mother but also to come into contact with the outside world, they will be unable to cope.[22]

The view of these 'professional outsiders' seems to carry not a little fear that the myths about the power of mothers to change the world might in fact be true. No threat of feminist revolt could surely be as disturbing as the actual possibility that mothers might, with quiet strength and determination, be able to create a qualitatively different kind of human being.

In terms of psychological theory, children who are secure and loved in their early years grow into secure and competent adults. If Maria's children are bound to become social casualties then this theory must be wrong. Maria's solitary achievement was not the product of some natural earthmotherly quality but of a carefully thought out and executed process. The task she embarked on was consciously chosen and in what she achieved she proved that 'good' mothering requires skill, strength, awareness and determination, qualities which are not normally regarded as 'feminine and maternal' as well as patience and love, which are. In her we can see a strong model of motherhood and one which can be respected, even if few of us have the temperament to copy her.

I have written at some length about external stresses which push us down at this vulnerable stage of mothering. We are told repeatedly that children who are secure and loved in their early years grow into secure and competent adults. Yet we see nothing dangerous in leaving that burden of responsibility for mental health on the shoulders of women who have to cope with hostility, indifference and virtual solitary confinement. Women can only provide love and nurture if they feel some love for themselves, some sense of worth. It is very difficult to value being female when your body is a badge of inferiority. It is very difficult to believe, amidst the jokes about tits and boobs and knockers that your breasts can provide milk enough to feed your baby. Amidst the stereotypes of earth mothers, blonde bombshells, neurotic housewives, liberated career women, it is difficult to find a place of rest, a sense of self, a semblance of dignity.

I have placed emphasis on these social stresses in the belief that the mountain of sand can be removed, or at least turned into a hill. Psychological stresses are more difficult to define and are often a result of insecure childhoods resulting from mothers being under stress. Unhappy children grow into unhappy adults and produce more unhappy children on and on down the generations. The problems inherent in trying to break this vicious circle have puzzled psychologists and psychotherapists for years. Certainly a system of child rearing which keeps mothers and children cooped up in virtual isolation does little to protect children from experiencing the full effects of their mothers' despair.

Most mothers are pressed down but not all become depressed. There are ways to cope with that mountain of sand, with help, and not all of us experience its weight and threat in the same way. We are, even as mothers, very different people with different values, expectations and needs; with different backgrounds and living conditions and with different children.

From the woman who finds immense pleasure and satisfaction in caring for small children to the woman who finds small children intolerable there is the usual curve of individual variation. What is considered normal or abnormal in that curve at any given point in history is purely arbitrary. Truby King's 'good' mother was a very different sort of person from the 'good' mother expected by today's popular psychologists.

When we are depressed and we feel guilty and failures, it is important that we seriously reassess our expectations of ourselves and ask whether we would expect so much of another woman. It is essential also to accept the reality of what we *do* feel rather than punishing ourselves for not feeling something else. The following story shows, I hope, that amidst all the blanket condemnations and judgements, there are those who care, who understand, who will help:

There was one mother with a toddler and a new baby and she'd come, it was her first visit with the new baby, to check that everything was going all right. Now the toddler was a sort of one man demolition unit. He went around, tipping over chairs, climbing on chairs so that you had to grab them before he tipped the whole lot over. Cups of tea were made and handed round and he *quite* deliberately knocked his mother's tea over on to the ground, then howled because he'd burnt his hand. She was very bright and very composed, really, considering the circumstances and I thought she was absolutely desperate. I said to the health visitor, 'She's got her hands full, hasn't she?' 'Oh yes,' she said, 'but she's a marvellous girl, copes with everything'; and I thought, 'Like hell she does!' And afterwards I went over to her and said, 'Do you find you get desperately tired at this stage with a toddler and a new baby because I just didn't know some days how I was going to physically put one leg after another, and just keep going.' And she sat down, put the baby in the carry-cot and burst into tears. Nobody else had asked her was she tired because she didn't say she was tired, she didn't look particularly tired. She was bright, she made a huge effort, she was immaculately turned out, the kids were immaculate. So she wept and I said, 'Look, I had a postnatal depression. I had a complete collapse, I felt I couldn't carry on, I had no help at all, so I *do* know what you feel and *please* accept that dozens of other people know what you feel *and* feel it too,' and she said, 'Oh, but I've got a marvellous husband and he does everything for me and I feel so guilty and my mother's been terrific . . .' and on and on. And I said, 'Will you please accept the fact that you feel like this. Once you've accepted it then we can do something about it.'

12. *Private and Confidential*

I remember sitting on the sofa facing the windows in a sort of heavy, lumpish haze. Autumn was coming on, the time of year Yorkshire folk call 'the back end'; the leaves of the massive plane tree outside were turning yellow-gold. Each falling leaf was a dead hope, the end of a possibility of better things. Unfelt tears trickled down my cheeks, a numb weeping.

Imogen was at her toddlers' club and Pippa slept; she was an angel child and never cried or fussed without reason. I felt doubly guilty about that, as if I deserved something more punishing from my baby for the incompetent way I was caring for her. She slept and I sat and watched the tree and my mind raced. Questions and answers, long monologues, conversations, storytelling, philosophical explorations endlessly worked in my mind. These long internal dialogues soaked up time and concentration to a point where it became almost impossible to concentrate on the most ordinary task.

I lifted a bucket full of dirty nappies into the sink to rinse them before washing and came back to reality with my hands freezing in the water. My watch told me I'd stood like that for nearly two hours. I went to the shops and stood facing rows of tins, unseeing, vaguely aware of people turning to stare. I tried to write letters and spent an entire evening writing one line. Like threading cotton through the finest needle's eye, the smallest action required immense efforts of concentration; *everything* required that kind of effort and I couldn't manage it.

Tears came easily but provided no relief because they were unfelt, they simply drained off energy like blood from an anaesthetized wound. I could tell when I was talking that I appeared fairly rational but it didn't tie up with the desperate feelings working underneath. The intellect disdained such things and attempted to function normally above it all. I blamed myself for everything. Self-hate hugged me so close there was no room for anything but reproach and guilt, guilt, guilt.

I fed the baby when she cried and she thrived on it. I have no idea how many feeds she had a day or how frequently. I simply didn't care. If she cried I put her to my breast and sat and gazed at those dying leaves. It's as well I was breast-feeding, I could never have sterilized bottles and mixed feeds. If I really worked hard I could manage to change her nappy but it didn't seem to worry her that she wasn't changed very much. She was a beautiful baby, sweet natured and unde-manding; I still marvel at that.

I had no real trouble sleeping but I didn't eat. Not, I think, because I wasn't hungry, but because I couldn't concentrate enough on preparing food. I was at my best in the morning and the depression worsened throughout the day. I certainly managed well enough to take Imogen to school and collect her but that was about all.

When did all this begin? I don't think there was a be-ginning in the sense of falling off a cliff; one minute on firm ground, the next crashing into blackness. It was more like one of those leaves, slowly and inevitably drifting down, down.

Maybe it started during pregnancy when I was so very tired and worried about the birth, or during the bleak and miserable hospital stay. I think all that contributed. But I was happy to be home and I was convinced that I would be fine once the baby slept through the night. I was very tired those first nine weeks with a new baby's routine to see to and a toddler to be given special attention. I coped beautifully. The flat was clean, the nappies washed, the food bought and pre-pared. I allowed myself no disorganized, sloppy behaviour as I had with the first baby; after all, I was an experienced mother wasn't I? I knew what it was all about:

I find *far* more people get a true depression after a second, far more. Just think of the two experiences. The first time, given that you've got a family, parents and in-laws – *everybody's* thrilled, you're having your first baby, they cluster round, they knit, they buy and there's terrific atten-tion and then . . . I've asked so many, dozens and dozens of women, 'What was the reaction when you told your

mother, your mother-in-law, the neighbours, you were having *another* baby?' They said, 'Oh, are you?' and that's it.
'Oh, Jane's having another baby' and the support from
family, the excitement, the interest, the moral support, isn't
there the second time because it isn't a novelty.

If you sit in the clinic you can spot the first timers because they're beautifully coiffured and wear make-up.
They've stepped straight out of the bath and spent two
hours getting ready to come, it's the highlight of the week.
The ones who've left the toddler, maybe with the neighbour, they look harassed and they're tired. They probably
had a fight with him to eat his lunch and get him in a clean
nappy before they handed him over. They arrive at the
clinic and they're worn out. The staff will say, 'Your first
dear?' 'No.' 'Oh well, you know what it's all about' –
now she may be the woman who is most under stress because she's got an eighteen-month-old, she's getting no
sleep, he's opening all the cupboards and pulling everything out. She needs more support than the first timer.

This is the view of one lay counsellor and she is correct in
that second-time mothers are usually neglected, expected
to cope easily, not assumed to have any problems of adjustment like first timers. Certainly the problems are different
but they are no less severe. The chief problem is learning
how to balance conflicting demands. Toddlers have a genius
for timing their potty demands *exactly* when the baby needs
feeding. Toddlers hate to have their old routine upset by
new babies and it is often unsafe to leave toddler and baby
alone in a room together. Nor do husbands always appreciate that two children create three times the work.

It is also useful to look for a loss situation in a depression. I shall write more about loss in the next chapter but in
relation to the birth of a second child, it is usually forgotten
that there is a significant loss of the special relationship between mother (and father) and their firstborn. I remember feeling quite desperate when I was in hospital after Pippa's birth
because I missed Imogen so much and no one seemed to understand. The focus of attention is usually on mother and baby,

not mother-baby-toddler which is a somewhat more complicated situation.

There is no way of predicting which women will be depressed after which babies. Some women are depressed after their first baby but not the second, some after the second but not the first, some after both. In one study of severely depressed mothers 49 per cent were first-time mothers.[1] In Pitt's study of less severe depression, however, there was no significant difference in parity (number of children) between depressives and controls.[2]

I came home from hospital with my first baby on Christmas Eve and we spent Christmas Day with friends. There was something magical about having a tiny baby at Christmas. I was very happy and despite all kinds of worries in the two years that followed I remained happy. I had the daughter I wanted and we suited each other very well. I had many good friends close at hand and a helpful husband. For the first time, and without clearly realizing it, I did less and less writing. I lived on the surface of things and neglected my inner world. By the time I became pregnant for the second time the neglect was showing; not only that, but my supportive environment was changing. It seemed about the time that Pippa was born, as though a storm passed through the group I had felt was so firm; marriages broke up, jobs were changed, people moved house. Emerging from a gruelling three days in hospital I arrived home to a harassed husband, a disturbed and demanding child and friends fraught with problems. The cocoon which had protected me from the bleaker realities of motherhood was torn open but I was not yet ready to fly.

The health visitor informed me that she wouldn't expect to see me at the clinic each week since I was obviously an experienced mother. When Pippa was about five weeks old Imogen got mumps and I had a sick little girl and a new baby. My husband started a new job and was absorbed in that. The only person who was aware there might be problems was my GP who asked me at my postnatal check if I felt depressed. I didn't. He explained that postnatal depression was very common and said I must go and see him if it developed.

It developed. Nine weeks after the birth, Pippa finally slept a full seven hours. I expected to feel very much better. I did not. My concentration fragmented and I was able to function very little. My husband became increasingly irritable and tense. He didn't realize what was happening and had a lot to cope with in a new job. He felt very hard-done-by that he was doing his best and had to come home every night to a miserable wife. I knew I was miserable. I tried not to be but I felt totally desolate. I felt that no one in their right mind would really want my company, so I shut myself away more and more and tried not to bother people. The feeling of abandonment was intense. There was no one to turn to who would provide comfort. I was alone. Yet I had a baby and a small child, so I was unable to be alone.

The kind of depression from which I suffered is sometimes called reactive. This means that a sense of loss experienced as a child is reactivated later in life by a similar set of circumstances.

In 1947, when I was six, my father took a job with Shell in Borneo and we all went out there for three years. There were no schools, so my mother taught us. She was the only mother in that little European community who bothered. When we returned to England we were put in boarding school and our parents returned to Borneo. I did not see my mother again for two years. Uncomfortably I straddled three worlds. I spent my holidays with my grandmother in her two-up-two-down cottage; a clean, shining and immaculate house with no hot water and a chemical lavatory down the back yard. I watched her washing with her dolly tub, posher and wringer, and ironing with flat irons heated by the fire. In term-time it was school uniform, the smell of polished wood floors, sleeping in dorms, prep and compulsory games. Letters would come from my mother who was living in a land where crocodiles floated on hazy jungle rivers and was sleeping at night under a mosquito net with the sound of casurina bugs outside, a land three thousand miles away.

I missed my mother very much. It was in these years that I started writing: bleak, desolate poetry was followed by novels and finally plays. Writing became my means of coping with a sense of not belonging anywhere, a means of trying to explore the painful connection between my inner world and outer reality. Writing became my solace and joy, an activity so intimately connected with my sense of self that I neglected it at my peril.

In a very interesting and simple piece of research conducted at St Thomas's Hospital in 1973 Eva Frommer and Gillian O'Shea set out to discover whether it was possible to identify mothers who might be vulnerable to depression by asking a group of married first-time pregnant women if they *felt* they had been separated from one or both parents before the age of eleven. The group of 'separated' mothers was then matched with controls, and follow-up interviews were carried out at three-monthly intervals during the first year of the baby's life. There was a marked increase of depressed mood among the 'separated' women which reached statistical significance about a year after birth. At this time 64 per cent of the 'separated' mothers appeared depressed to the interviewers, though they did not report depression, as compared to 34 per cent of the controls. The total figures here are again high. Of eighty-nine women interviewed a year after the birth, a total of forty-four were observed to be depressed, almost 50 per cent.[8]

Since a number of 'separated' mothers did not become depressed and a number of 'non-separated' mothers did, we cannot consider childhood separation to be anything more than a predisposing factor, though an important one. It is another fragment in that stained glass window.

Frommer and O'Shea comment in their research that the behaviour of the 'separated' women to their infants seemed to be more readily polarized into either over-anxiety to be a 'perfect mother' or lack of care, than that of the controls. Dana Breen, in her research into well-adjustment to motherhood, again with a group of first-time mothers, makes a similar comment:

At the same time as they found themselves in greater conflict with the image of the perfect selfless ideal mother they described, the ill-adjusted women were less able to admit to imperfection when the focus was on motherliness ('maternal dimension') specifically. It is as if they had a stricter idea of what they should or should not be like and that what they should be like was more unattainable than the other women.[4]

She made no study of separation in childhood but notes that of the ill-adjusted group, eleven out of thirty-nine had lost one parent as compared to only one of the well-adjusted group, numbers which are too small to lead to any conclusions. These two pieces of research both seem to show that, with first babies at least, women who believe in the popular image of the perfect selfless mother and try to conform to it are those who may have had upset childhoods and are likely to be vulnerable to depression.

Whilst I don't see this internal idealized picture of the perfect mother as part of my own depression, I believe the effect of false expectations can be devastating. I certainly expected myself to be able to cope with two children as easily as I had with one. In fact I expected more of myself as an 'experienced' mother than I had as an inexperienced one.

I also see that the regimented treatment I received in the hospital postnatal wards could easily have reactivated feelings I had at school. At school there was no alternative but to obey rules and accept blame. There was no one to turn to for comfort except friends within the system. I have always, in consequence, turned to female friends for support and comfort in times of crisis. After Pippa was born they all seemed to be involved in crises of their own. I tried to start writing again, usually after the two a.m. feed which was the only time there was, but I was too exhausted.

Most cases of postnatal depression occur within two to three weeks after birth but there are a significant number which start later, as mine did, at two, three or even six months after the baby is born. There is no obvious explanation for this. It is often very difficult, anyway, to say exactly when a feeling of general exhaustion and discontent becomes a clinical depression. In my case the loss of concentration was probably the most significant thing.

One day I went shopping and crossed the road at a particularly dangerous junction. A car came whizzing round the corner and swerved to miss the pram. I walked home shocked. I put the baby in her basket and walked round and round the room. I knew I needed help. I had endangered the baby. I wasn't functioning. The baby needed someone else to keep an eye on things.

It is difficult to admit even to yourself that you are unable to cope with a situation you feel should be well within your capabilities, let alone admit it to someone else. Despite this, a part of me recognized that something had to be done and because my GP had asked me to see him if I was depressed, I was able to locate what was wrong. I eventually telephoned the surgery after it should have officially closed and was allowed in. My doctor's receptionist was a friendly dragon-at-the gate and ran a flexible appointments system which for me, at that point, was invaluable. I suspect that had I been given an appointment for the next day or the day after that I simply wouldn't have gone. As it was I didn't want to go.

I telephoned a woman I had only met once and asked her if she would collect Imogen from the toddlers' club. She was immediately sympathetic and offered to look after the baby as well. These two immediate responses to requests for help were very important.

My doctor was concerned about my condition but not surprised by it. He explained to me that postnatal depression was very common. He believed that the birth of a baby represented a family crisis and that when things went wrong it was usually the woman who broke down first because women had to carry the most stress. He didn't feel this indicated it was solely the woman's problem, however; he felt that husbands were under stress too, though often refusing to recognize it. He told me that drugs would help to relieve my symptoms but would not remove the causes of the depression and recommended that I accept a referral to the Marriage Guidance Council, if possible with my husband, whom he said he would also like to talk to. I was surprised by this suggestion since it seemed to me self-evident that I was the problem not the marriage. However I was grateful to be given any possible alternative to drug treatment.

It was a long consultation and I left with a feeling of being cared for, as well as with a prescription for anti-depressants. I contacted the Marriage Guidance Council and while I was waiting for an appointment I saw my doctor, briefly, every other day. My husband agreed to counselling though only, initially, because he thought it would help me.

I had an exceptionally good doctor. Not all GPs are as aware and concerned about the problem as he was. Some don't seem to be aware of it at all: 'The trouble is that I am very depressed. I told my doctor, and he said, "Whatever for?" '[5] Others, who are aware of the problem, tend to treat it with drugs alone: 'My GP did not say very much to me at all. He listened, handed me a prescription and told me that it would be some time before I got better and asked me to go back when the tablets were finished. The second visit was similar.'

But there seems to be in addition a heartening number who, despite their heavy workloads, manage to offer something more than little white tablets:

> He somehow conveyed the feeling that help was there, he was there, which is what you need. Not only was he there, the surgery was there, help was down the road. He was an enormously humane man.

> She was really good, she was ever so understanding. I told her how things were between Steve and myself and I said about our sex life: She immediately said, 'Right, let me examine you,' and she examined me and she said, 'Well, it's healing now, but you are just too tired, you're worn out.' I said I was at my mother's. She said, 'All right, I'll put you on to tablets as long as your mother'll look after the babe.' So she gave me tablets which knocked me out for forty-eight hours. The doctor knew all about my father dying and everything else. She said to me I just had too much to cope with anyway, the upsets we'd had . . . Then we left the baby there one weekend and we came back here so *we* could talk things over on our own. That again was at the advice of the doctor which was one of the good things about her.

Which kind of GP a depressed mother finds herself talking

to and what kind of treatment she receives is really a matter of luck. Since good doctors have as heavy, if not heavier, workloads as those who rely on dishing out pills or the 'pull yourself together' routine, it seems reasonable to assume that the heavy workload argument is used as a convenient excuse by those who dislike this aspect of medicine. It is, in a sense, the way the doctor protects himself from demands which he may feel unable to meet. Doctors are trained, after all, to diagnose and treat physical illness. They do not receive case-work or counselling training and without that kind of skill it is difficult for them to know what kind of help they can provide other than drugs.

We were always promised that with lighter workloads the maternity services would provide better care. We were always promised that with fewer numbers or more teachers, classes in our schools would be smaller and our children would receive more attention. The birth rate has fallen from around 750,000 babies a year in 1962 to 596,000 a year in 1976. As a result the services have actually deteriorated. Small, local, maternity units are being closed all over the country, ensuring that pregnant women have to travel much farther in order to wait the same length of time for the same brief consultation. Primary schools are closed as rolls fall, teachers are unemployed and small children have to travel farther to sit in the same-sized classes as before. This leads me to conclude that a large drop in the number of GP consultations would lead, not to more and better attention, but to shorter surgery hours and the closure of small practices. We would then have farther to travel for the same service we have at present.

Good doctors always seem to manage somehow to provide enough help. It is difficult because GPs are expected to provide a great deal of support without receiving much themselves. Social workers and counsellors have regular meetings to discuss their case-loads and share and investigate problems; doctors have no such opportunity unless they work in large group practices. Whilst condemning the authoritarian doctors whose prejudice against women does untold damage, we must not forget the pressures suffered by others: 'That particular doctor committed suicide, a tragic thing, he knew what it was like to be depressed and I think that's possibly why he was so good.' Doctors have a higher suicide rate than any other professional group and it is thought that those most at risk work in general practice.

I imagined that a marriage counsellor would be a cosy, well-meaning woman, very sympathetic and ready to give good advice, rather like the 'aunties' of the agony columns. I don't remember very much about the content of my first interview, I was so low, but I do remember the powerful presence of a calm, still woman who gave no advice at all but asked some disturbing and difficult questions.

I tried to take the drugs, but after two days I was so dopey I couldn't do anything and I nearly dropped the baby when I was feeding her. I flushed them down the loo. My husband arranged for me to go away and stay with some old friends in Newcastle. I took the baby with me and Imogen went to stay with her granny. My friends lived in a house which looked out over water which I found strangely comforting. The company of relaxed, accepting friends, the change of scene and relief from a part of my responsibilities helped enormously.

The worst of the depression lasted no longer than seven or eight weeks but I was still prone to depressive mood swings for a long time after that. It took a year before I felt confident that I had emerged from that narrow, suffocating tunnel. For the whole of that year we continued to go for counselling every week. We seemed to be on an emotional see-saw. As I improved, Richard sank down. He too was very depressed for a short time which proved my doctor's diagnosis of family crisis correct.

There is no evidence to suggest that fathers suffer from postnatal depression. In that men experience less direct stress, change and exhaustion than their wives after the birth of a new baby, it seems reasonable to expect them to cope better. The concerned father is under some pressure, however, because a new baby inevitably causes an upheaval. If he has to cope with any other major changes, he too may suffer: 'It was an extremely difficult time for us because my husband resigned from his job shortly after the baby was born, so he was depressed as well. We were sort of propping each other up.' Trying to cope with a depressed wife can, in itself, prove a tremendous strain: 'It was only when I was ill that he started getting down. If I'd been able to stand it, he would have been all right. Also he was here on his own, I was at my mother's with the babe and he was missing us like heck because it was very difficult for him to get over.'

As far as my children are concerned it is impossible to say what effect this year of crisis has had on them. They are both much loved and cherished and we can only hope that this present and continuing love will heal any wounds and help them to grow into strong, self-confident women.

For myself, I have learned, slowly and painfully, to recognize that I have needs which must be satisfied if I am to grow and develop. One of these is the need to locate and express anger. Another is the need to employ my talents usefully.

'Depression is the aching of an unused talent.'[6]

13. *The Black Rose*

The black rose blooms and we know postnatal depression means mothers in despair; energy gone underground, flatness and greyness above ground; desolation, silence, withdrawal from life. Women have described this variously as being behind a black curtain, falling into a black pit, walking through a tunnel, falling into darkness. It is like the night of the soul, the extinguishing of a flame. How the baby perceives this withdrawal as the cloud moves over the sun, we can only guess.

When we lose something that is important to us, we grieve for it. It seems curious to consider having a baby in terms of loss when the gain of the baby is the most obvious part of the experience. The gain of a baby brings with it, however, loss of independence; loss of habit; loss of routine; loss of pregnancy; loss of old family relationships; loss of sleep. There is a great deal of change which occurs at the very point when a baby first enters the world.

The loss of status, independence, money and perhaps professional identity which occur with the birth of a first baby, hit some women harder than others. A woman who is used to having an active and responsible role to play in the outside world may experience considerable conflict when she becomes that social nonentity, the housewife. The beautiful woman whose self-esteem is constantly boosted by male admiration may feel a similar conflict when she has to spend the bulk of her time with other women and small children. The woman who is used to being treated like a child and having decisions made for her may find the responsibility of a baby's welfare terrifying.

However much she wanted her baby, a woman can feel the loss involved in change keenly and feel guilty about it. Some women find it so intolerable being at home all day with a small baby that they have to return to work in order to cope at all. These women inevitably feel guilty because all 'good' mothers are supposed to want to stay at home with their babies and to enjoy doing this.

The 'bad' mother is selfish, harsh and uncaring; the 'good' mother is warm, comforting and giving. These images crop up so frequently in the literature connected with child rearing and are so generalized that I suspect that they are derived more from unconscious feelings than from common sense.

Jung believed that there are elements in all of us which belong to a collective unconscious, i.e. which are part of our human heritage and can be found in all human cultures as symbols or archetypes. One of these archetypes is the Great Mother, a primordial image containing both comforting and devouring qualities; the witch and the goddess; the loving and the terrible. Jung recognized, however, that although aspects of the archetype influenced the psychological development of individual women in different ways, no human mother could possibly be expected to carry the full burden of such unconscious projections. In his book *The Archetypes and the Collective Unconscious* he warns of the dangers:

A sensitive person cannot in all fairness load that enormous burden of meaning, responsibility, duty, heaven and hell, on to the shoulders of one frail and fallible human being – so deserving of love and indulgence, understanding and forgiveness – who was our mother. He knows that the mother carries for us that inborn image of the *mater natura* and *mater spiritualis*, of the totality of life of which we are a small and helpless part. Nor should we hesitate for one moment to relieve the human mother of this appalling burden, for our own sakes as well as hers. It is just this massive weight of meaning that ties us to the mother and chains her to her child, to the physical and mental detriment of both.[1]

The moral exhortations and moral judgements laid on mothers seem to be more connected to unconscious feelings connected with the archetype of the Great Mother than they are to the actual lives and living conditions of ordinary human mothers. The image of the selfish, 'bad', uncaring mother comes through in this kind of statement: 'Although there are advantages to the breastfeeding mother none of them is powerful enough to influence a mother who is only concerned with her own wellbeing';[2] whereas the human reality of a woman who ignores her own wellbeing can look very different to the fine image of the 'good' mother we are supposed to imagine:

> I tried to feed him and he'd keep pulling away from me, it was a definite rejection and it was all my own fault, I could see it. I was making it worse for him by carrying on feeding really. I was very guilty. I felt awful, I really did feel guilty about it and the more guilt I felt, the more I tried to feed. I shouldn't have done, I should have just given up and put him on the bottle. People felt they were being kind and they said to me, 'Oh, you should carry on breast-feeding, he's been so tiny, he's had a bad start, give him the best.' So I did and I hated every minute of it. I really got to hate breastfeeding.

By being caught up in the unconscious projections connected to the archetype of the Great Mother, human mothers easily lose all sense of their own individuality and worth. They are stretched to fit impossible expectations and forced to cut off their own needs. Women who have a strong sense of individuality and worth escape the rack but the most vulnerable easily start to disintegrate. The most terrible loss of all is the loss of self.

Depression isn't like measles. It doesn't have a set incubation period or a definite pattern of symptoms. It doesn't run any set course and then vanish. Women experience depression in different ways and it is not always easy to say at what point a feeling of being low, tired and fed up with the world turns into an 'ill' depression.

In order to try and make some sense of the mood disturbances they have to deal with, psychiatrists classify depression into different types. Some psychiatrists believe the various types of depression are different and separate entities, others that depression is a particular mood which simply varies in individual cases from the fairly mild to the very severe.

Anxiety, grief and sadness are not in themselves abnormal emotions. Anxiety over unusual events alerts us to the possibility of danger; grief is an inevitable result of our ability to love; sadness is the natural risk of seeking happiness. It is when these moods become excessive either in intensity or in duration that they are seen as unhealthy. Since some people live life far more intensely than others anyway, our normal personality also has to be taken into account.

It is usual to describe three kinds of depression occurring after birth: 'the blues', postnatal or 'atypical' depression and puerperal psychosis. Whether these are in fact different types of reaction or simply represent different degrees of severity is a matter of opinion.

There is usually a feeling of anti-climax after any dramatic event. Add this to physical exhaustion and the soreness of stitches and it is not surprising that so many women feel physically and emotionally wobbly after having a baby. There is also a very dramatic change in hormone levels after birth which I shall talk about in Chapter 15.

'The blues' or 'the weeps' are very common in the week or so after birth (see Chapter 6). What usually happens is that there is a tremendous feeling of elation after delivery and for a day or so after birth. This is followed by a period of great emotional vulnerability. Small things like a husband or friend being late at visiting time or reading a sad story in a newspaper can set off a flood of tears. There may, in addition, be good cause to cry, if the baby is ill, for example, or the hospital staff are unpleasant.

Some women suffer more from 'the blues' than others and some don't suffer at all. It is unpleasant and upsetting to be so vulnerable and weepy but fortunately the mood lasts for only a couple of weeks at most. If it continues for longer, it probably means that it has turned into something more serious.

There has been so little research into the milder forms of postnatal depression that no one knows what connection there is, if any, between them and 'the blues'. In some women 'the blues' may be fairly mild in hospital, clear up completely, and then a depression may start four or five months later: 'I had the weeps but not deep depression, you know, the awful owl that sits there. I got that afterwards.'

Some women become depressed who don't suffer from 'the blues' at all.

Postnatal depression is the term popularly used for those kinds of depression which are mild enough to enable women to continue functioning somehow but severe enough to make them feel that life is pretty dreary and intolerable. This state is sometimes called 'atypical depression' because it differs in various ways from 'classical' (or typical) depression or 'neurotic depression' because anxiety can be the most pro- nounced symptom, or 'reactive depression' because the mood is a direct reaction to stress such as ill health or deformity in the baby, bereavement, separation, complete physical ex- haustion; or the mood may be a reactivation of a sense of loss experienced earlier in life.

Whatever its label, depression still hurts. Some women feel much happier if they have a name for their mood, others hate being labelled. Hanging a label on women trying to cope with a crisis can be dehumanizing. The most important thing is to be able to recognize and accept that the mood exists in the first place.

The main symptoms include despondency; tearfulness; feelings of inadequacy and inability to cope – especially with the baby – other women seem to be managing so well; feel- ings of guilt, especially over not loving the baby enough; unusual irritability, adding to feelings of guilt; loss of appe- tite sometimes leading to anorexia – the inability to eat; loss of sexual interest; hostility or indifference towards a normally loved husband; extreme anxiety over health, the baby's, hus- band's or own; sleep problems, usually difficulty in getting to sleep at night (when the baby is *not* crying); nightmares; fear of leaving the house (agoraphobia) or attacks of panic when out, for example whilst shopping.

Thankfully no woman will suffer from all these symptoms but even having two or three of them can be a very nasty experience. The combinations vary with different women. For some, guilt may be the most obvious:

I just couldn't understand it but I just felt so guilty because, you know, I felt I was no good as a mother, I felt I couldn't cope with the baby, I felt I was letting my husband down, I felt I was letting the family down, I wasn't feeding the baby properly and, of course, all this time my milk was getting weaker and weaker because I was tired.

Others experience the mood as something much more physical:

To me it was a physical depression as much as anything, you feel very slow, very heavy. Aggravation, irritation and a great feeling of, what's the word psychiatrists always use – persecution, very, very strongly. The great persecution feeling that *everybody* was against me and *nobody* understood me at all, that was very strong.

Others feel intensely anxious:

One lunchtime my husband's car broke down and as he couldn't let me know I became convinced that he had been in an accident. After that I could hardly bear him to be out of my sight. I was convinced he was going to die. I cried all the time, clung to him and wouldn't plan for the future or even lay the table for two in case he never came home. I went to the doctor having got to the stage when I thought that I might as well kill myself as I couldn't face life without my husband who was wonderfully loving and patient throughout.

Or simply inadequate:

Her crying made me worse and it became a vicious circle. After about four weeks I began wishing I had bottle fed her and at five and a half weeks I put her on the bottle. I became very depressed and when the baby cried, I cried. I hated my husband to go out of the flat (an upstairs flat in a heatwave is not the ideal place!) and I was really scared of the baby. I didn't feel any strong maternal feelings until she was about four months old. This also worried me – I thought I was rejecting her. Eventually I went to see

the doctor . . . I think the tablets helped but I was eager
to get back to work – anything to get out of the flat.

Postnatal depression may start two or three weeks after
birth or two to six months later. It may last for only a few
weeks or it may drag on for years. It is thought that it occurs
in about 10 per cent of women though the figures may be
higher.

Women who suffer from postnatal depression are unlikely
to have any previous psychiatric history. In Pitt's study, three
depressives and six controls had a history of previous psychiatric illness and two from each group had previously
suffered from postnatal depression.[3] Dalton found no difference in the incidence of previous psychiatric illness between
women who became depressed and those who didn't. She
found that the women who became depressed after birth
were those who had no pregnancy symptoms, were anxious
during the first three months of pregnancy but elated for the
last six months and were very keen to breastfeed. She believes
that the findings point to a hormonal explanation of post
natal depression.[4]

Puerperal psychosis is much rarer than postnatal depression
and much more severe. It occurs in about 1 in 500 newly
delivered mothers, though estimates vary. There have been
many studies of these psychotic conditions, chiefly because
women who suffer from them usually require hospitalization
and are therefore easier to study. Puerperal psychosis take
different forms though studies show that between 60 per cent
and 67 per cent are depressive. Psychotic depressions are so
severe that very often mothers cannot function at all. Some
times a mother may be so paralysed by her fear of hurting
the baby or so guilty about her own badness that she may kill
herself and her child.

Other psychotic reactions may be either manic, with symp
toms like suddenly spending far too much money, talking
endlessly, sleeping little or cleaning the house at two a.m
manic depressive where there are wild variations in mood
from high to low; or schizophrenic which involve delusions
particularly about the baby, hearing voices or sometimes see

ing things. Some of the symptoms in psychotic states may be present in milder forms of postnatal depression. A condition is usually called psychotic when it is so severe that the woman appears to be out of touch with reality. Psychiatrists generally agree that psychoses which occur after the birth of a baby are no different from those which occur at other times of life.

One woman I talked to described her psychosis as more of an anxiety state: 'I went completely out of my mind in the sense that I thought the baby was dead and I thought I was dying as well. It wasn't a straightforward depression. I wasn't crying all the time or anything. I just couldn't eat, couldn't sleep and couldn't get out of my mind that there was something wrong with him. Eventually I just thought he'd died and thought I was dying as well.'

And another described an experience of schizophrenia: 'I had sort of elation, what they call schizophrenia. I wasn't depressed at all. I was anxious at times and I was very elated and had a lot of delusions about all sorts of peculiar things. It was as though I just couldn't organize myself to do anything. I couldn't concentrate. At one stage I thought the bomb had dropped. We lived in the middle of a very small town and on Sunday morning there was nobody about. I got up one morning and I was just convinced that everybody was wiped out and we were the only ones that were left. I thought it was quite exciting, actually, it was a challenge. I wasn't frightened.'

It is not possible to predict which mothers will suffer from a breakdown and which will not. Some women who suffer from puerperal psychosis have never suffered from any mental disturbance before and have no desire to ever again. There is a one-in-five chance that a woman who has suffered from a psychotic breakdown with one pregnancy will suffer again with the next, but that statistical fact is no help at all in predicting in individual cases. For the woman who has suffered from a psychotic breakdown, the decision as to whether to risk having another baby is a bit like Russian roulette. Since stress factors are undoubtedly important, preparing a really secure environment might help to lower the odds.

In one study of puerperal psychoses there were six mothers

who had adopted babies.[5] This is not really so surprising since the desire to have a child has little to do with a woman's ability to cope with the stress of rearing it. I spoke to one mother who had suffered from a prolonged postnatal depression after adopting a baby. She claimed that many women she knew who had adopted babies had suffered from bouts of depression. She felt that adoptive mothers are given far too little help and preparation. The baby arrives and they are simply left to cope: 'We had no health visitor, nobody came to visit us. If I hadn't had good friends I would have had a complete breakdown. I had a great friend who lived nearly opposite who'd had three under five and she was wonderful. She came across and bathed Jane. She showed me how to do everything.' She didn't seek any form of help because she felt too guilty and ashamed at being unable to cope when she had chosen to adopt a baby:

> I was always so tired. I used to feel about ninety. I really felt a terrible failure all the time. As a friend of mine said, you had the double guilt. She felt the sadness of it all because of their parents. I must admit I didn't feel that so much but I felt we'd chosen to do this, we ought to be doing it doubly well. I ought to be doing it twice as well as any other mother. I felt all the time that I wasn't doing it well enough. I should have been not only a good mother but a super mother because we were lucky enough to get this good little girl. Everybody kept telling me how lucky I was and I felt like saying, 'Why don't I feel I'm lucky?' I used to go to bed at night and think, perhaps it's a ghastly dream and I shall wake up and find it never really happened.

It is thought that about 1 in 2000 women suffer from post-adoptive depression though, obviously, there are many who remain unnumbered because they struggle through on their own without seeking help. The fact that women become depressed after adopting babies is often used as an argument for seeing postnatal depression as being caused by stress rather than hormone imbalance. That stained glass window, however, has many pieces and each picture has a different composition.

In his book on human aggression Anthony Storr devotes a chapter to describing the way in which depression is connected to problems in handling aggressive feelings. He comments that neurotic women tend to be aggressive and that 'The neurotic man is, as we have said, less than normally aggressive. This simply means, of course, that his aggression is repressed, and is apt to show itself either in unreasonable bursts of irritability, or else in moods of depression which, . . . are intimately connected with difficulty in handling aggressive feelings.'[6] In view of his belief that women are 'naturally' less aggressive than men – or should be – it is not surprising to find that he fails to point out that depression is overwhelmingly a female complaint. Twice as many women suffer from depression as men and virtually all advertisements for mood-altering drugs in medical magazines show a miserable woman. It is women who have the greatest difficulty in handling aggressive feelings, chiefly because it's not supposed to be feminine to have them. The old nursery rhyme tells us

> What are little girls made of?
> What are little girls made of?
> Of sugar and spice and all things nice
> That's what little girls are made of.

Whilst I appreciate that it must be most unpleasant for little boys to be told they are made of slugs and snails and puppy dogs' tails, at least it is not an image which follows them into adult life. Unfortunately this is not true for adult women who are supposed to remain permanently sugary and nice. An angry woman is a shrew, vixen, virago, hell-cat or fishwife, all just about equally unpleasant figures.

Little boys are expected to be dirty, noisy, boisterous and aggressive. Little girls are expected to be clean, calm, quiet and unaggressive. I have heard my own little daughter being told off by another woman at the age of *three* because 'little girls don't have their vests hanging out of their trousers'. By preventing little girls from attacking their physical environment and learning how to stick up for themselves we manage to communicate to them that only by being continually placating, pleasant and compliant can they hope to be loved. If a mother behaves in this way herself the teaching is doubly reinforced by example.

There is, in addition to this kind of upbringing, the disturbing fact that our culture still assumes that both parents would 'naturally' prefer sons:

> *Traditionally* women want a boy, but this is not always the case. There are instances where *some* women have a strong desire for a girl . . .
> *Occasionally* the woman herself may be happy to have a child of either sex, but her husband for a variety of reasons, may strongly desire one particular sex, *usually* a boy.[7] [My italics]

If mothers traditionally want sons and fathers usually want sons and only some women occasionally want daughters there must be millions of baby girls who grow into the world knowing that they are, by virtue of their sex, their very bodies, a disappointment to their parents, second best, second choice.

Thus the cultural inferiorization of women has been both reflected in and perpetuated by the family and demographers worry that if parents are ever able to choose the sex of their children there will be an imbalance of males in the population. As women grow in self-confidence and learn to value their abilities and potential, it is likely that far more will positively desire to have daughters and a normal curve of individual variation should establish itself in sex preference of children.

As far as postnatal depression is concerned neither the sex of the baby nor the desired sex appears to make any difference. Pitt discovered that in his group eighteen depressives and fifteen controls had boys and of eight depressives who admitted a sex preference in pregnancy, four had babies of the sex preferred, a proportion which was identical to that of the controls.[8]

The effect on female psychology of the traditional preference for sons is, I suspect, very considerable. If a girl feels she cannot be fully loved for what she is, her self-esteem must be damaged. One young mother said to me in the maternity ward, 'Mine is a girl, but I don't mind *really* because you can dress 'em pretty.' It seemed to me a tragic commentary on the female condition.

If more daughters than sons feel fundamentally inferior they are more likely to develop depressive characteristics which are easily hidden in their traditional role. By altering the sex in the following passage, which I have done by adding brackets, we can see how this happens:

> The conviction of being fundamentally unlovable, so characteristic of depressive people, does not make a man [woman] an agreeable person except superficially. For he [she] will be so hungry for love, and so frightened of appearing assertive or in any way aggressive that he [she] will submerge his [her] own personality in that of the other, and use his [her] capacity for doing this as a kind of blackmail. In the end this manoeuvre defeats its own object for one cannot love someone who hardly exists in his [her] own right, and excessive sympathy, however welcome temporarily, soon becomes as intensely irritating as frank dependency of which this is a distorted form.[9]

Since women have traditionally been encouraged to be completely dependent and to submerge their personality in that of their husbands and children and have, indeed, been positively discouraged from being people in their own right, it is hardly surprising to find that depressive characteristics and the traditionally approved female personality are virtually identical.

Learning how to recognize and express anger creates very great problems for many women who have repressed their rage for so long that it seems as though it no longer exists. Advice to mothers has traditionally included the repression of anger: 'And remember, an "atmosphere" is as bad as a row in its effect on the young. So if you love your child and want him to grow into a mentally sound and healthy adult, remember the old adage about the soft answer turning away wrath, and pray (and work) for peace in your home.'[10]

This kind of moral exhortation (and blackmail) presupposes that anger repressed will simply cease to exist. It won't. Anger which is denied a proper outlet either turns into self-hate and aggression against the self or it explodes in childish and sometimes violent forms. All close relationships are ambivalent. We often resent the most those we love the most. Children loathe their parents at times and parents loathe their children. The guilt connected with this resentment is only present because we have been led to believe that love excludes all bad feelings. It doesn't. If our children can learn to tolerate ambivalent feelings we shall have given them far more than by attempting to avoid an 'atmosphere'. Dr Spock's advice is considerably more realistic: 'It helps to clear the air for everyone to admit that fights are one of the facts of life, even among grown-ups, that people can fight at times and still love and respect each other, that a fight doesn't mean the end of the world.'[11]

Anger, loathing and aggression turned against the self in a depression can be very severe: 'We had one girl who cut herself, nicked herself all over with a razor blade, none of them sufficiently deep to kill her; she just methodically and carefully nicked herself at half-inch intervals everywhere so that she was streaming with blood.' This kind of self-hate can end in the complete destruction of the self in the form of suicide. By refusing to admit to resentment and angry feelings because, perhaps from childhood, we have learned to feel they were bad, we push them out of conscious knowledge where, like any fearful thing they grow into immense proportions. Depressive people very often have a terror of the devastation which they might cause if they released their anger yet do not hesitate to attack themselves. During the violence of a depression it is always better to turn anger outwards. Admitting to angry feelings makes it much easier to deal with them without violence. Self-assertion is a proper use of anger, and learning to be angry instead of hurt when we are belittled is, especially for women, an important step away from depression.

Postnatal depression is not a new condition. Hippocrates cited the case of a woman who gave birth to twins, developed rest-lessness and insomnia on the sixth day after birth, became delirious on the eleventh day and went into a coma and died on the seventeenth day. He was of the opinion that blood collecting at the breasts of a woman indicated madness.[12]

It is only recently that depressive illness after childbirth has been isolated from mental disturbance by physical in-fection. Before the discovery of antibiotics, ECT and the main tranquillizers and anti-depressants, many women died from puerperal psychosis. The causes of death were toxaemia, de-hydration, starvation and suicide. At St Nicholas Hospital, Newcastle-upon-Tyne, of 134 women suffering from puerperal psychosis who were admitted between 1927 and 1961, four-teen died, but of these, thirteen were admitted between 1927 and 1941.[13] The incidence of puerperal psychosis appears to have remained fairly static for the past hundred years or more which has led some psychiatrists to wonder whether the cause may not, in fact, be hormonal (see Chapter 15).

The milder forms of postnatal depression have been re-searched very little, even today, and there are no figures at all for earlier times. 'The blues' was first mentioned in medical literature in the late nineteenth century and was sometimes referred to as 'milk fever'. Whether we live in a more or less depressed state than our mothers or grandmothers is there-fore anyone's guess. One woman summed up very well the problems involved in depending on the memory of older women:

My mother-in-law, who is now elderly, was a midwife in the 1920s and 1930s and both she and her contemporaries say that they never experienced any depression themselves nor did they ever see any cases of it. Obviously this is either true or not! If it's not, then one assumes that mothers did get depressed, but were not clinically recognized and were just told to pull themselves together – or one could assume that they have forgotten much of their experiences, and would have regarded depression in themselves as a sign of weakness and not to be admitted.

Certainly working women who lived through the appalling

hardships of the Victorian and Edwardian eras worn out by constant childbearing, poverty and physical hard work had very good cause to be depressed. Since there was, until very recently, considerable fear and superstition about mental disorder, however, and no effective treatment for depression, we shall never know how many women coped because they had to and how many failed to cope at all.

The law has recognized for some time that women may become emotionally disturbed after the birth of a child. The Infanticide Act of 1938 states that a mother cannot be found guilty of murder if she kills her own child within twelve months of its birth, provided 'the balance of her mind was disturbed by reason of her not having fully recovered from the effect of giving birth',

It has never been easy at any stage of history to admit to mental disorder in the family. In the 1970s we hope that we are more enlightened in our attitudes but there is still a great deal of prejudice. The fact that so many studies indicate that women do not go for treatment when they become depressed shows that either someone is failing to recognize what is happening or is unwilling to try and do anything about it. In a study of medicine takers, prescribers and hoarders in 1972 Karen Dunnell and Ann Cartwright discovered that adults seemed less likely to consult their doctors about depression, persistent headaches and acute sore throats than doctors felt appropriate.[14]

Part of the reason why women may not consult their doctors when they are depressed after aving a baby is probably because they don't recognize they are. Eva Frommer and Gillian O'Shea discovered in their study that nearly 50 per cent of the mothers observed to be depressed by experienced social workers didn't report feeling depressed.[15] One of the features of a depression is that it makes the world look so grey that it often seems as though everything around you is going wrong and that you are to blame for it. In this state it is really very difficult to stand back and assess your own mood, especially if you hav never suffered from depression before. For those women who are aware of their own mood, there is the problem of admitting to their feelings. Depression is a sign of weakness, failure, inability to cope, it is something that happens to other people: 'I imagined a rather temperamental, rather stupid, rather dull woman bursting into floods of tears.'

It is very difficult in these circumstances to seek help: 'The trouble is that people like me who are lucky enough not to suffer postnatal depression are either unaware of it, or somewhat superior because we have escaped it. Those who do suffer it are so withdrawn and often so guilty about it that the help intended for them (such as it is) never reaches them.' Often it is only when the situation reaches a crisis point that a woman really accepts that something is wrong and needs attention:

As I say, me and my husband had this row over absolutely nothing. There was definite tension between us. Our sex life was absolutely nil because I was too damned tired for it. Also I had problems then that it hurt me because the wound didn't heal. In the end I took the baby for a walk and I ended up at my mother's house, and she lives eighteen miles from here. I walked there and my husband didn't know where I was. I realized when I got to Mum's that it must be me, I must be ill.

Accepting that we feel really low; accepting that we not only find it hard to cope but that we don't really want to cope; accepting that 'I can manage' is more often an expression of hope than a statement of fact; accepting that caring for a small baby is not always the most enjoyable task in the world though it has to be done; accepting that we *are* tired and need a rest; accepting that we are more important than the housework; accepting these things without guilt can be the start of recovery: 'The important thing was to admit it, but I wouldn't really admit it then because I felt so guilty about it, I felt I shouldn't have felt like that.'

We know very little about the relationship between mothers and daughters. Theology, art, sociology and psychology have told us only about mothers and sons and fathers and daughters. This is not surprising since it has been sons and fathers who have shaped our culture and our ideas. In folk-culture, however, the defensive and cruel jokes of music-hall comedians about wives and mothers-in-law point to a closeness between mothers and daughters which men find threatening. There is also the old saying that

> A son is a son till he takes him a wife,
> A daughter's a daughter the rest of her life

which reflects the woman's central place in the family with men seen as important only in terms of the woman they are attached to, be it mother or wife. This is a curious reversal of the more usual view of women being important only in relation to the man they are attached to, be it father or husband.

In that mothers, daughters and sisters often form a very close network, especially in the working-class extended family, it is possible to see something of the kind of close attachment and support that women can provide for each other, a closeness which is often greater than that between husband and wife.

The first intense love relationship a female makes is with another female. The closeness and mutual identification between mother and daughter is permitted because it is not seen as dangerous. An equal closeness between mother and son would be considered unhealthy. Mothers communicate to their daughters the nature of the female condition in everything they do and in everything they are. This is a heavy responsibility as Adrienne Rich points out:

What do we mean by the nurture of daughters? What is it we wish we had, or could have, as daughters; could give, as mothers? Deeply and primally we need trust and tenderness; surely this will always be true of every human being but women growing into a world so hostile to us need a very profound kind of loving in order to love ourselves. But this is not simply the old, institutionalized, sacrificial, 'mother-love' which men have demanded: we want cour-

ageous mothering. The most notable fact that culture im-
prints on women is the sense of our limits. The most
important thing one woman can do for another is to
illuminate and expand her sense of actual possibilities. For
a mother, this means more than contending with the re-
ductive images of females in children's books, movies,
television, the schoolroom. It means that the mother herself
is trying to expand the limits of her life. *To refuse to be a
victim*: and then go on from there.[16]

There is much work to be done in exploring all the implications and possibilities which exist in the relationship of
mothers to daughters. It is, perhaps, at the time of birth,
when we become mothers ourselves that we become most
aware of our close connection through flesh to our own
mothers. It is at this time that we need to be connected to
and cared for by women; not necessarily our own, biological
mothers, but women who will provide for us a protective
magic circle so that we can make the transition from daughter-
hood to motherhood which I suspect needs to be made anew
after each birth. The experiences of women I talked to varied,
but most felt the need for another woman's presence in the
weeks after birth:

I've been very much closer to my mother since I've had
children than I was before. I just felt a terrific need for
her – because I thought possibly she was the only person
who would be able to tolerate my acute involvement with
myself both before the baby was born and after. There
were also overtones of being able to lean totally on somebody else's shoulder.

You need a mother, yes you do, you need a mother to say,
'You're all right, you're doing jolly well.' I had my mother
for about four days and then she went teetering back home
absolutely worn out.

It depends entirely on what your relationship's like with
them really. It doesn't change because you have a baby.
I was really glad to have my Mum. The only thing that

marred it was the fact that my husband didn't want her to be there.

I suspect there is a confused identification which occurs to a degree in all mothers after birth between themselves and their own mothers. It is perhaps in women who have suffered the most loss in their childhood that this confusion is most apparent. The psychiatrist Dr Desmond Bardon has written in an article on puerperal psychosis: 'A woman who in early childhood had serious difficulties in her relationship with her mother may, when she herself becomes a mother, recreate, by her inappropriate responses, the same situation between herself and her child. She sees her mother in herself and herself in her child.'[17] He believes that anxiety and depression can follow as a result of this kind of disturbed relationship. He treats his patients in a mother-and-baby unit where he encourages the nurses to provide woman-to-woman support:

> An essential part of the treatment situation in such a unit is the close proximity and availability of the nurse to give help, support, encouragement, advice and to immediately take over the baby from the mother when she feels she cannot cope with it or tolerate it. The nurses must be aware of their own maternal feelings and be prepared to encourage the mother to take back the care of the child again as soon as she is ready.[18]

He states that by using this method, 'Some 42 per cent of the last 70 cases of puerperal depression admitted to our mother-and-baby unit recovered without any anti-depressant medication or ECT after an average stay of 4.2 weeks.'[19]

It is worth remembering that emotional deprivation is not simply a result of poor mothering. It occurs when a mother dies, it occurs when children have to be taken into care, it occurred on a massive scale in the last war when thousands of children were evacuated from the cities and sent to live with strange families in the countryside.

There are some men who are capable of providing warmth, food and comfort but on the whole the nurturing role in our society is carried on by women. The adult female population is expected to provide care for children, old people, sick people, and men. Caught in this situation, the new mother exhausts herself caring for her baby, her children, her husband and her home and caring less and less for herself. So who mothers mothers? Increasingly the answer seems to be the drug company Roche Ltd. Of the ten million tranquillizers and anti-depressant tablets taken in Britain every day, seven million are swallowed by women.

14. *Talk and Tablets*

Throughout history and in most cultures, madness has been taken as a sign that a person is possessed by evil spirits and has been treated as such by priests and witch doctors. Until the present century madness and sin have been seen to walk hand in hand; indeed the whole area of mental health is one where the ideas of guilt, punishment and reparation still thrive. Since insanity, like crime, disturbs the orderly working of society, the insane, like criminals, have traditionally been beaten, locked away, restrained by straitjackets, chains and padded cells and forgotten about.

At the end of the eighteenth century doctors began to take over the role of priests in the treatment of the insane. Asylums were established in Europe and scientific studies of various forms of mental disturbance were carried out. The subject was still surrounded by much popular superstition however, and it was possible for the Victorian medical profession to terrify several generations by claiming that masturbation led to insanity.

In the twentieth century science has taken over from superstition in the treatment of mental disorders though there is still a great deal of fear and condemnation in the community. As late as 1955 a sentence of two years' imprisonment was imposed for an attempted suicide which was varied on appeal to one month. It was not until 1961 that the Suicide Act changed the law so that it was no longer a crime to kill yourself.

Psychiatrists have fought a consistent campaign to persuade lay people to regard mental disorder as an illness, a sort of disease of the mind that needs medical attention rather than a punishing evil spirit which needs exorcizing. Just at the point when the community seemed to be accepting this view of things, an attack was launched within psychiatry itself against what was called the 'medical model' of mental disorder. The critics of the medical model claim that psychiatrists simply suppress symptoms and return patients to the same intolerable conditions which produced the symptoms; that they act as agents of the state by altering or containing socially undesirable or embarrassing behaviour instead of helping people to extend the possibilities of their lives. The anti-psychiatry view is that the insane are people trying to find a way to cope in a mad world. Those who adapt to intolerable and unhealthy social conditions are crazier than those who mentally rebel and retreat.

Certainly the medical profession has always been very conservative, and doctors have traditionally tended to treat patients in such a way that they will conform to the accepted norms of society. Thus behaviour which is not socially approved, like homosexuality, is treated as mental illness until society decides to be more tolerant. There are more extreme examples of this process:

It is, of course, nothing new for doctors to turn behaviour they disapprove of into illness . . . Dr Samuel A. Cartwright in his 'Report on the Diseases and Physical Peculiarities of the Negro Race', published in 1851 in the then prestigious *New Orleans Medical and Surgical Journal*, described the new disease of drapetomania. This disease he named from 'drapetes', meaning a runaway slave, and 'mania' meaning madness.[1]

Since no one knows what causes depression or schizophrenia, the two major mental disorders, social, psychological and medical theories all manage to co-exist amongst those who work in the mental health field. This can be rather confusing for people who suffer a breakdown and simply want help.

Many women who suffer from postnatal depression manage to pull through simply with the help and support of friends and relatives, people who are prepared to be with them and share the crisis. This is the kind of community support which has always had a great part to play in the prevention and alleviation of emotional distress of any kind. Beyond this there are many different specialists who study the psyche and it is useful to know who does what.

Obstetricians have no real interest in postnatal depression and they know very little about it. Obstetricians like to think that having babies makes women happy and prefer to ignore the fact that it makes large numbers miserable. There is little point in asking an obstetrician for advice at a postnatal visit unless he is exceptionally sympathetic.

Most women who suffer from postnatal depression are treated by their general practitioner in a more or less sympathetic manner and probably with drugs. A good GP will try to organize some kind of human support in addition. If a GP intensely dislikes dealing with emotional states and weeping women or if he feels a depression is particularly severe, he will refer the mother to a psychiatrist.

Psychiatrists are all doctors of medicine (as opposed to doctors of philosophy) and are the only practitioners in the mental health field who require a medical degree. Psychiatrists usually work in hospitals and treat patients either as inpatients or as out-patients like other medical specialists. Psychiatrists do not have to go through any form of personal analysis before they are allowed to practise. Apart from a few exceptional cases the National Health Service will only pay for treatment given by a GP or a psychiatrist. Any other treatment has to be paid for privately.

Psychologists take degrees in psychology which is the study of human motivation and behaviour. Psychiatrists conduct research into mental disorder, psychologists conduct research into human behaviour. Psychologists work in virtually every field: educational psychologists study how and why we learn; industrial psychologists study how and why we work; child psychologists study how children develop. Only clinical psychologists treat patients, though psychological studies may influence the way in which patients are treated.

Psychoanalysts treat patients or analysands and usually need a degree in psychology. Psychoanalysts follow the methods of mental analysis advocated by Freud which include intensive probing into childhood experiences and dream analysis. Psychoanalysts are not allowed to practise with patients until they have been through a course of analysis themselves. This can mean three one-hour sessions a week for up to four years so it is not only a very lengthy process but at £10 to £15 a session, a very expensive one.

Jungian analysts who follow the methods advocated by

Jung have much the same kind of training as psychoanalysts. Analysis by any method is lengthy and expensive and is often used by those who feel they would like to lead a more productive life rather than by those who are in the throes of a mental breakdown and want a speedier kind of treatment.

Psychotherapists could be anybody. There is nothing to stop you, me, or the milkman from setting up shop as a psychotherapist and there has been some concern expressed by doctors about this. It is unwise to go to a psychotherapist without a recommendation from someone you trust, unless they belong to a reputable school of psychology. Many psychotherapists are trained and controlled by reputable organizations and the training is much the same as that of analysts. The human growth movement of the early 1970s produced a crop of new therapies: Gestalt; transactional analysis; primal therapy; encounter groups and so forth. Most of these have something of importance to offer and all have to be paid for privately.

The majority of women who suffer from postnatal depression cannot afford private therapy even if they are attracted to the idea. Those who see a specialist almost invariably see a psychiatrist.

Psychiatrists work in strict geographical districts so it is really a matter of luck what kind of psychiatrist a woman comes into contact with and there is little chance of going to a different one without moving house. Most psychiatrists rely on physical therapies like drugs and ECT (electro-convulsive therapy) though some attempt to investigate emotional problems may be made as well. Any form of psychotherapy takes time, however, and psychiatrists have very heavy workloads so that there is a limit to what they can offer: 'He came to my house which was civil I suppose and he offered a fair amount then I think, but it's in the nature of what they're up against; they can only offer emergency care really.'

There is also the danger when time and attention are limited that patients will exaggerate symptoms in order to appear more interesting:

He was asking me a lot of questions which were obviously set questions, I felt as if he was ticking off the symptoms.

He asked, 'Do you hear voices?' and at that time I said yes, I had this thing that when I turned the radio on I heard space remarks and moon messages which went when I turned my earrings off. I think I made that up, actually, on the spur of the moment.

The relationship between male psychiatrist and female patient, like all such medical relationships, tends to be authoritarian and thus reinforces feelings of helplessness and compliant behaviour which are unhelpful to women, though they may be approved socially. In that psychiatry provides an emergency service, however, the physical treatments offered can be effective.

People who suffer from severe psychotic depressions are often treated by electro-convulsive therapy. This form of treatment consists of passing limited electric shocks through the brain. No one understands why it works but it has been found to be effective as a treatment for depression. The worst side-effect is memory loss which can be considerable in some cases: 'If it happened again I would try and not go back to hospital because of the loss of memory, it makes you lose your confidence. I couldn't even remember how to cook or just how to run a house. It was quite hard to get back into the swing of things.' Psychiatrists vary in the extent to which they use ECT and some have been accused of being rather too liberal in their use of it. Others use ECT only in very extreme cases and prefer to rely on drugs.

It is only in the last twenty years that tranquillizers and anti-depressant drugs have provided the possibility of relieving the suffering which is the main symptom of depression. These drugs have been so successful that they are increasingly used to treat not only clinical depression but a wider and ever-widening range of personal and social problems. It is, after all, much easier to keep mothers with small children in poor housing permanently sedated rather than have to re-house them. In Aldous Huxley's *Brave New World* the entire population was kept docile and happy by being fed a mood-altering drug, 'soma':

'My dear young friend,' said Mustapha Mond, 'civilization

has absolutely no need of nobility or heroism. These things are symptoms of political inefficiency. In a properly organized society like ours, nobody has any opportunities for being noble or heroic . . . The greatest care is taken to prevent you from loving anyone too much. There's no such thing as a divided allegiance; you're so conditioned that you can't help doing what you ought to do. And what you ought to do is on the whole so pleasant, so many of the natural impulses are allowed free play, that there really aren't any temptations to resist. And if ever, by some unlucky chance, anything unpleasant should somehow happen, why, there always *soma* to give you a holiday from the facts. And there's always *soma* to calm your anger, to reconcile you to your enemies, to make you patient and long-suffering.'[2]

Huxley wrote this in 1931 before the tranquillizing drug industry had even started but he understood that absolute political control would depend on ensuring that people loved their servitude. He comments that, 'Round pegs in square holes tend to have dangerous thoughts about the social system and to infect others with their discontents.'[8]

In Britain, approximately £12,000,000 is spent annually by the National Health Service on mood-altering drugs and one journalist has estimated that at the present rate of increase the year 2000 will coincide with the total tranquillization of America.

As far as postnatal depression is concerned, however, drugs can mean the difference between sinking and swimming. Whilst social and personal problems should always be given attention, there is not always an obvious and immediate solution to them and meanwhile a mother has to cope with her baby. Personal crises which follow the birth of a baby are especially difficult to cope with simply because there is no time to be alone.

Both tranquillizers and anti-depressants act by altering the brain's chemistry. Stress can alter this chemistry and so can mood. Fear and anxiety trigger stress hormones which produce a chemical chain reaction round the body affecting appetite, sleep patterns, heart rate, sexual functioning, etc.

Whether the hormones trigger the mood or the mood triggers the hormones is something of a chicken and egg debate but certainly body chemistry and psychological state interact. Drugs work on this interaction by putting the body's chemistry back into harmony and thus altering the mood. Talk therapy on the other hand aims at treating the psychological state which will then automatically correct the body's chemistry. Drugs tend to work rather faster but they can have unpleasant side-effects.

Drugs always have different effects on different people. Some people become physically dependent on psychiatric drugs and suffer from withdrawal symptoms when they stop taking them. Some people become psychologically dependent and find it difficult to cope without them, much like alcohol or tobacco. The following is a brief list of the psychiatric drugs which may be prescribed for women suffering from post-natal depression. Which drugs or combination of drugs are prescribed will depend entirely on the doctor's clinical judgement.

The minor tranquillizers (these are largely Benzodiazepines) are Valium, Librium, Nobrium, Mogadon, Serenid and Ativan. These drugs are used mainly to suppress anxiety and tension. Common side-effects include: drowsiness, dizziness, apathy, fatigue, confusion, lapses of attention, shakiness and unsteadiness of movement. Less common side-effects include: diarrhoea, constipation, headaches, rashes. Librium may markedly stimulate the appetite. Sometimes these drugs actually increase tension and produce aggressive outbursts.

Anti-depressants fall into two groups, the monoamine oxidase inhibitor (MAOI) group and the tri-cyclic group:

Tri-cyclics: Tofranil, Anafranil, Amitriptyline, Prondol, Surmontil, Lentizol, Prothiaden, Dothepin.
MAOIs: Parnate, Nardil, Marplan, Actomol, Niamid.

These drugs are used to help lift a depressed mood of misery and hopelessness accompanied by sleep problems, poor appetite and other symptoms of depression already mentioned (see Chapter 13). The main effects of the drugs are to improve appetite and sleep, lift the mood of misery and reduce anxiety. The problem with anti-depressants is that they don't have any effect on mood for about two to three weeks though the side-effects are present from the start.

The most common side-effects are: dizziness, drowsiness, a dry mouth, confusion, sweating, shaking, racing heart, blurred vision, constipation, skin rashes, delay in urination, weakness when rising from a prone position and increased weight because of water retention. The effects of other drugs such as alcohol may be increased.

Very dangerous side-effects can result from taking the MAOI group together with certain foods. The combination can produce very high blood pressure which shows itself in severe headaches, breathlessness and palpitations. Some of the foods to be avoided are: cheese, Marmite, Oxo, Bovril, all yeast foods, alcohol, chicken liver, game, yoghurt, broad beans and bananas. All other drugs should be avoided including cough mixtures, nasal inhalants, suppositories, and local and general anaesthetics. Most doctors warn their patients about these dangerous side-effects and a chemist should provide a list, but I have heard of cases where this hasn't happened.

For many women who have to cope somehow with a baby to care for and a house to run, these side-effects can prove too much to cope with. Whether a woman continues to take anti-depressants for the recommended period depends on how disabling the depression is, how severe the side-effects are, whether there is help available in the house and how worried the woman is about becoming dependent on drugs. Most women do not like the idea of taking mood-altering drugs for any length of time and I suspect that millions of pounds' worth of drugs are flushed through the nation's sewers annually: 'I went to see the psychiatrist a few months after and he said, "You're all right now, but continue to take the drugs for six months," and I just stopped then, because I was fed up with taking them. I was still depressed.' This woman obviously preferred the depression to the drugs. Other women find the drugs don't have very much effect:

I didn't like the idea of taking drugs, I got off them as

quick as I could. I was off drugs by the time the baby was six months. I couldn't see what good they were doing me and there was no difference when I stopped. Obviously you have to withdraw them gradually, I didn't just stop taking them or anything like that. I reduced the dosage, but it was on my initiative.

However, anti-depressants can be a useful prop to help mothers survive a difficult period in their lives: 'I started anti-depressants almost immediately which I think was a good thing, they do work. They make you feel peculiar but they do make you feel physically better quite quickly actually, they positively lift your mood, it's quite uncanny.' Whilst a bottle of tablets is a poor substitute for a hand in the dark, they can help to provide a breathing space so that personal or social problems can be assessed and necessary changes made where possible.

Most forms of talk therapy aim to help people resolve unconscious conflicts by becoming more aware of their feelings. The most revolutionary of Freud's discoveries was the existence of the unconscious or subconscious mind which revealed itself through dreams. Freud believed the subconscious was a kind of quagmire of repressed sexual desires. Jung, who originally worked with Freud, broke away from him because he saw the unconscious as something more creative. Jung believed that the unconscious mind contained primitive archetypes which revealed themselves in dreams when areas of the personality were being neglected.

Many other psychologists have developed, adapted, and added to the theories of these two great founding fathers of psychology, but the recognition that there is a huge area of human experience and feeling which exists beyond conscious thought has significantly altered the way in which we view human personality and behaviour.

What is unconscious is, by definition, unknown. Speculating about other people's unconscious fears, desires and motives is a favourite game for amateur psychologists (and some professional ones!) but it doesn't prove anything. When researchers talk about unconscious anxiety or unconscious rejection of pregnancy/motherhood/femininity or what you will, they have left the realms of science and are simply guessing.

Psychology is not an exact science; the irrational nature of the unconscious mind sees to that. Nonetheless, psychotherapy can be helpful in enabling us to recognize and accept what we really feel rather than pretending that we feel something else. We develop our patterns of thinking, feeling and behaving from childhood and we get so used to them that most of the time we are not aware of what we are doing. People who break down during a crisis in their lives, or people who feel they have problems coping with life at any time, often seek help from psychotherapists in an attempt to understand their problems and hopefully change their behaviour.

Changing behaviour and patterns of thought and feeling is very difficult and only a little success can be expected at any one time. Many people have believed they have become changed people as a result of a particular therapy, only to discover that old habits die hard and old learning is stronger than new learning.

One of the dangers of psychotherapy for women is that it may be used to adjust them back into the stultifying maternal and feminine role against which they are rebelling. No therapy worth the name should limit human growth and development but Freudian based therapies especially have been accused of doing this to women. Germaine Greer assesses the problem thus:

The essential factor in the liberation of the married woman is understanding her condition. She must fight the guilt of failure in an impossible set-up, and examine the set-up. She must ignore interested descriptions of her health, her morality and her sexuality, and assess them all for herself. She must know her enemies, the doctors, psychiatrists, social workers, marriage counsellors, priests, health visitors and popular moralists. She must analyse her buying habits, her day-to-day evasions and dishonesties, her sufferings, and her real feelings towards her children, her past and her future. Her best aides in such an assessment are her sisters.[4]

This assessment is accurate in the sense that women are unlikely to grow and develop as people without radically analys-
ing their domestic situations. If other women are available
to lend support, this may be enough, but a good therapist
ought to be working on the same lines.

Women who suffer from postnatal depression and who
can afford the time and the money to see a psychotherapist
may find the exercise useful. There will, however, be no
more guarantee that it will be successful in removing the
depressed mood than drugs would be. The advantage of talk
therapy is that it pays attention to the problems that lie behind the depression, which drugs don't. This assumes that
postnatal depression is a kind of mental rebellion against intolerable pressures which many cases undoubtedly are but
some cases are not.

Each woman has some intuitive idea whether she would
find a talk therapy helpful and there is no earthly use in
going for this form of therapy if you don't really believe in it
and aren't prepared to work hard at it. Since most forms of
psychotherapy are expensive they will be out of reach of the
majority of mothers anyway. There are voluntary organizations, however, which can offer help.

The Samaritans have captured in their name the caring and
befriending nature of the organization. As names go it is
difficult to think of anything more patronizing than the
Marriage Guidance Council. It summons up the image of wise
elders in council guiding the ignorant young through the
hazards of marriage. There have, it is true, been several attempts to change the name, none of them successful, which
means that few people realize that the Marriage Guidance
Council provides a comprehensive counselling service for
the single as well as the married, homosexual as well as hetero-
sexual and one or both partners in a marriage.

Counselling is a less concentrated form of psychotherapy.
The art of good counselling is not to give advice but to help
people become aware of the ways in which they think, behave
and feel, thus enabling them to see how their relationships go
wrong. Because the work is voluntary most of the counsellors

are women which makes a change since 85 per cent of psychiatrists are men. There is also a reasonable chance that a female counsellor will herself have children and will therefore have a working knowledge of the stresses and problems involved in babycare. These things are not supposed to matter in good counselling, but I am convinced they do.

Most husbands fight shy of going to counselling, but that need not matter. Nor does a woman need to be referred by her GP. She can make an appointment on her own. Counsellors are very carefully chosen, thoroughly trained and closely supervised so there is a fair chance that the exercise will prove helpful.

Marriage counsellors have been accused of trying to keep bad marriages stuck together and encouraging women to conform to the traditional feminine and maternal role. There may well be counsellors who try to do this but it is certainly not the purpose of counselling. Many couples go for counselling in order to be able to separate without bitterness and thousands separate without even considering counselling. And I can only say from my own experience that my counsellor seemed more concerned to see me moving outwards into the world than to see me reconciled to a life devoted to husband and children.

Because so many therapies have failed to come to terms with women's real problems, two female psychotherapists have set up a Women's Therapy Centre in North London which is run on a voluntary basis. The centre has a one-year waiting list which is an indication of demand for this kind of therapy. In an interview one of the therapists explained:

The woman I saw this morning had been in and out of hospital for seven years with anorexia and finally someone told her to come here. She had been pushed into hospital and pumped full of food and then released and told she had a disease. The point is, she had never been listened to. It's a good example of what women's therapy is about. We can help with her real fears about becoming a woman, being an adult. The treatment she had just further infantilized her – not being allowed to be in control of her own food. There is a contradictory message here: 'Be a big girl, but you can't really look after yourself.' It's a message women get in society.[5]

Therapists with a feminist perspective are more likely to take women's problems seriously and to work in an informal way as compared to the kind of authoritarian systems which male therapists use. Hopefully the idea of women's therapy will develop and centres will be set up in other parts of the country.

Many women have no desire to probe their psyche, they just want a helping hand for a few weeks, someone to share their problems, maybe take the toddler out occasionally or do a bit of shopping until they get on their feet. This kind of befriending is what the extended family and the close community has always provided. Since these are breaking down, organizations have to be formed to do the job.

Health visitors can help and some run SOS groups of mothers to help out in times of emergency: 'We started SOS groups, they're help groups for people who are wanting bureaucratic help or jobs doing and very often people with young babies need help for a period and then are very pleased to provide the same for somebody else.' Health visitors are, in fact, in the best position to detect and watch over depressed mothers and some are very concerned about the problem. Pitt comments that his research was suggested by a health visitor who commented on the frequency with which she found newly delivered mothers to be depressed and her request for guidance as to why this happened and how to give help.

Many health visitors, however, seem to be mainly concerned with the physical aspects of baby care and provided the baby is not actually neglected assume that all is well. Since many health visitors don't have children and many mothers have smiling depressions, this is perhaps not surprising; but it deprives depressed mothers of their most obvious source of help.

Apart from the mother-to-mother help organized by health visitors, if it exists, there is also help provided by voluntary organizations. The National Childbirth Trust runs postnatal support groups for newly delivered mothers, many of which

16

have experienced lay counsellors who can help those who are depressed. Lay counsellors have no formal training as such, but plenty of experience and should always know their limitations: 'The only thing that I let guide me is when I feel that anything I can offer is inadequate, is not going to be sufficient, or, having offered it, after a few weeks find that there's no difference, no improvement. I couldn't tell you how many people I've referred on.' Samaritans are lay counsellors in the same kind of way. They follow certain guidelines but their essential work is befriending, listening, caring.

Finally, for those women who are aware of suffering from depression, there is the self-help group Depressives Associated. This is an organization which was set up to enable depressed people to meet and help each other. Because there is a great deal of ignorance in the community about depression, it can be very therapeutic just to meet other people who understand how you feel. Contrary to popular assumption, depressed people are not depressing as a group and can give each other a great deal of help and support.

The two main risks of postnatal depression are that mothers will attack themselves or their children. The patience threshold in a depression is very low and mothers can easily lash out at their children in desperation and then loathe themselves even more for doing it. This doesn't mean that depressed mothers don't love their children – they usually love them very much – but simply that they are unable, for a time, to tolerate their demands or supply their needs.

Many mothers who have suffered from depression have felt that from the point where the baby was born they were seen to have no importance other than in relation to their baby. Often if postnatal depression is discussed at all it is in terms of the effect a depressed mother has on her baby and her family. That the mother is a suffering human being who is a person worthy of concern in her own right should never be forgotten.

15. *All Those Damned Hormones*

Puberty, childbirth and the menopause are all times of enormous social, psychological and physical upheaval when women are especially vulnerable to breakdown. Twenty per cent of acute hospital admissions are for overdoses, chiefly young women aged between fifteen and twenty-five swallowing mouthfuls of the very pills intended to make them tranquil. Depression is the most common complication following birth and depression often accompanies the unpleasant hot flushes, sweating and palpitations of the menopause.

In addition to these three major times of change, women also have to cope with the monthly rhythms of the menstrual cycle which can bring their own problems. Some women do not have periods at all (amenorrhoea), many suffer from period pains (dysmenorrhoea) and it is estimated that 40 per cent of women suffer from the premenstrual syndrome. This includes symptoms such as migraine, asthma, water retention, acne and general lowered resistance, as well as irritability and mood swings occurring in the few days before and the few days at the start of the monthly period.

Psychological explanations are often given to explain menstrual problems, usually along the lines of failure to adjust to the feminine role or, more recently, by Penelope Shuttle and Peter Redgrove,[1] as the result of the repressions and taboos placed on menstruating women.

During puberty, menstruation and pregnancy, after birth and during the menopause, however, there are fluctuations in the body's sex hormones and there are some doctors, notably Dr Katharina Dalton, who believe that it is the way in which the body adjusts to these hormonal changes which causes both menstrual problems and postnatal depression.

All bodily functions are regulated by hormones which are chemical messengers travelling on set routes through the body. If there is a shortage or an imbalance in hormones the body will react by producing either physical or psychological symp-

toms. The two female sex hormones are oestrogen and progesterone. These regulate the menstrual cycle, ovulation, pregnancy and the supply of breast milk.

Dr Dalton is a gynaecological endocrinologist, which means
that she specializes in the study and treatment of hormone-
related disturbances in women. She has been working in this
field for twenty-five years and is convinced that postnatal
depression is caused by the problems experienced by some
women in adjusting to low levels of progesterone after birth.

During the normal monthly cycle and for the first six weeks
of pregnancy progesterone is produced by the ovaries. Between the sixth and sixteenth week of pregnancy a new,
large factory, the placenta, goes into production and much
higher levels of progesterone are pumped into the body. Progesterone is nature's tranquillizer and high levels present in
the body may be one of the reasons why some women feel so
placid and cow-like during pregnancy.

With the delivery of the placenta, its hormone production is
cut off abruptly and there is no more progesterone in the
body until two weeks before the first menstruation. This means
that the body has to adapt itself to a sudden and considerable
chemical change. Since different placentas produce different
levels of progesterone the degree of adaptation will be different after each birth.

If a woman suffers from postnatal depression there is a
90 per cent chance of the premenstrual syndrome subsequently
developing. It would seem that some women, after having a
baby, have difficulty in adjusting to the permanently low
hormone levels of the non-pregnant state.

It is therefore possible to argue that a depression which
starts soon after birth becomes at the time of the first period
a part of the premenstrual syndrome and the mood simply
continues month after month for years. On the other hand
a depression which starts after birth may lift when the first
period arrives. Some depressions may not start until the
time of the first period when they become a part of the premenstrual syndrome. Since stress increases the symptoms of the
premenstrual syndrome, all the stresses surrounding the birth
of a baby would simply make the depression worse.

There are also some women who may become depressed

when they stop breastfeeding because they retain high levels of another hormone called prolactin. This can be diagnosed by taking a blood test and specifically treated with bromocriptine.

Dr Dalton claims that postnatal depression can be treated very effectively with progesterone which is a natural hormone as distinct from progestogens which are synthetic hormones. In her book *The Premenstrual Syndrome and Progesterone Therapy* she devotes a chapter to the differences between progesterone and progestogens, differences which many doctors do not seem to realize. She writes: 'Both are valuable in therapeutics but they are not interchangeable and progestogens are not just a convenient synthetic oral substitute for progesterone, and they should have no place in the treatment of the premenstrual syndrome, or the maintenance of pregnancy.'[2]

Progesterone cannot be taken in pill form. In order to be effective it has to be given as an intramuscular injection or in the form of suppositories (vulgarly known as bum bullets) or pessaries (inserted in the vagina instead). Progestogens are contained in the contraceptive pill but progest*ogen* lowers the blood progest*erone* level, which may be why women who suffer from the premenstrual syndrome become depressed, irritable and lethargic on the pill. Given this effect, it is obviously not sensible for a woman suffering from postnatal depression to take the pill. A diaphragm, cap, condom or sheath might be a better contraceptive to use, at least until the depression has lifted.

Dr Dalton suggests that postnatal depression should be treated by daily injections of progesterone until the initial symptoms have gone, which will probably take a few days. Thereafter suppositories should be used until menstruation returns.

The side-effects of progesterone are weight gain, usually in under-weight women, or weight loss, usually in over-weight women. Some women find they feel more sexy with progesterone therapy and others lose interest in sex. No drug interactions have been noticed with progesterone. There are forty women who have been on continuous progesterone therapy and under constant surveillance for ten years without suffering any adverse effects. Progesterone aids breastfeeding whereas anti-depressants can inhibit breastfeeding. Since you cannot take an overdose of suppositories progesterone is not danger-ous and women who have just had a baby are used to very high levels of progesterone.

One of the exciting possibilities of progesterone therapy is that it may be used as a preventative treatment for women who have already suffered from a severe depression after a pre-vious birth. If progesterone is given during delivery and con-tinued for a month or so afterwards, a depression may be avoided. This seems to offer real hope to those women who would like to have a second or third child but are too fright-ened of risking another depression.

Despite the fact that progesterone appears to be a very use-ful physical therapy for women suffering from postnatal depression, very few women receive it. This may be partly due to the fact that progesterone is a natural hormone and therefore cannot be patented, so it lacks the commercial promotion which drug companies usually give to their pro-ducts. Many GPs are suspicious of new hormone therapies, however, since there has been so much trouble with the old ones. Most psychiatrists do not accept that postnatal depres-sion is caused by hormone imbalance though some are inter-ested in the idea. The author of an American book on post-partum psychiatric disorders has commented:

It is quite possible that the very common syndromes of lesser magnitude are sequels to physiological disturbances. Despite severe limitations in knowledge regarding basic mechanisms of pathological psychophysiology there are some promising leads towards therapy. The first of these was the demonstration by Blumberg and Billig that progesterone was effective in preventing relapse.[5]

And an English psychiatrist, Dr Colin Brewer, argues that psychotic reactions after abortion being only one-fifth the rate of those after birth, may point to biochemical changes being an important factor in the cause of postnatal depres-sion:

Although it is possible that abortion is only one-fifth as stressful as childbirth, I think that unlikely. Furthermore, most women who have children are very happy about it, while even in these enlightened days you don't hear about abortion parties. It seems, therefore, that the excess of puerperal illness probably reflects the biochemical and hormonal changes which are almost certainly less profound after abortion than after childbirth.[4]

Dr Brewer is at present conducting research into hormonal levels after abortion and after birth.

No physical therapy should be considered to be enough on its own for any form of postnatal depression, since women always need support. However, as physical therapies go, progesterone would appear to have advantages over anti-depressants in that it has fewer side-effects, it works faster and cannot be taken as an overdose. It is to be hoped that once the medical profession are satisfied with its effectiveness and safety it will be made more widely available to women.

The fact that progesterone has been an effective therapy for many women suffering from postnatal depression does not necessarily prove that depression after birth is caused by hormone imbalance.

Dr Dalton's research into postnatal depression at the North Middlesex Hospital revealed that the characteristics of women suffering from postnatal depression were different from those which might have been expected. Depressed mothers had welcomed pregnancy, were free of pregnancy symptoms and were enthusiastic about breastfeeding. They were anxious in the first three months of pregnancy but very happy for the rest of their pregnancy, and depressed after the birth. She argues that these mood swings in women who welcome pregnancy are caused by a reaction to marked differences in hormone levels at different stages of pregnancy and following birth.[5]

Nothing is ever absolutely true of all women and some of the women I have talked to felt ill during their pregnancy and were depressed afterwards. However, many women feel their depression is something very physical and Pitt comments that one woman in his study described her symptoms as like the premenstrual tension syndrome. Most doctors appear to agree that 'the blues' is probably caused by the body readjusting to hormonal changes, which is one of the reasons why weeping women in postnatal wards aren't taken very seriously.

Indeed the danger of seeing postnatal depression as solely caused by hormone imbalance is that this can lead to its being dismissed as trivial and unimportant, the frequent fate of so many 'women's problems'. One woman I talked to told her obstetrician at her postnatal check that she felt depressed. 'Don't worry,' he said, 'it's your hormones'; and sent her away to live through six months of isolated 'hormonal' misery. Whatever its cause, a depression is a frightening and dangerous experience and a depressed mother always needs care and support in addition to physical therapies.

Since we have very little understanding of how psychological states and body chemicals interact there can be no definite conclusions as to the cause of postnatal depression. Further research into all aspects of the subject is much needed. Obviously the effect of hormonal changes cannot be overlooked, but neither can all the other factors which I have discussed in this book:

I think the hormonal changes have a large hand in it, they're extremely significant. I think past history, past life, your attitude to having a child, the stimulus of your marriage or your set-up with your boyfriend are obviously relevant, as well as the degree of immediate support afterwards, or lack of it and your own expectations about yourself.

16. *In Conclusion*

The fact that motherhood drives many women to despair is so disturbing and threatening, that the lack of literature on the subject of postnatal depression is perhaps more revealing than surprising. It is a common human reaction to hope that by ignoring a problem it will just go away.

When a personal problem is shared by a large enough group of people, it becomes a social problem. When a third to a half of mothers with pre-school children have been found to be significantly depressed over a twelve-month period we are faced with a problem which can no longer be ignored.

It is alarming that this situation has been hidden for so long and that so little has been done to investigate it. Thousands of women become distressed and unhappy as a result of having a baby; some of them suffer for years, neglected and dismissed.

The only comprehensive book in world literature on psychiatric problems connected with childbearing was published in 1858;[1] the milder forms of postnatal depression have hardly been studied at all. Obstetricians appear to have little interest in the subject and psychiatrists consider that it does not exist as a special problem. Yet the figures insist that the bearing and rearing of children in this society endangers the mental stability of many women.

I have tried to show how and why this may happen by pointing out the multitude of pressures and the magnitude of change which the newly delivered mother experiences. Some of these stresses are inevitable, for the birth of a child is a momentous human event; but in the proper order of things birth should be a victory, not a defeat, and mothers should be esteemed, not despised.

Mothers embarking on the immensely complex and responsible task of child rearing do so without any social support. Our faith in the natural ability of our bodies to give birth to and feed our baby is consistently undermined, and our highly developed practical and intuitive skills in child care are dismissed as 'instinct'. We are told we are important but everywhere find we are a nuisance. Our small children are of little concern to any public authority; we are not expected to share either the pleasures or the strains of rearing them.

The nuclear family of mother, father and two or three children which is so convenient to an economy requiring a mobile labour force is one of the worst possible units for rearing the small children who will be the future labour force. It is simply too small; it is too private; there are no spare resources to rely on in time of emergency; there is no protection for children against their parents' violence. The baby reared by an isolated mother receives the magnified intensity of her every mood; if her mood is depressed, how does the child interpret it? What effect does it have on a growing mind to be exclusively in the company of a tired, unhappy mother?

In that it is possible, given the will, to reduce many of the stresses experienced by mothers, we should press for change. For example, home confinements must remain a safe option for women who want them; a system of maternity aides should be introduced to ensure that mothers manage to get enough sleep during the weeks after birth; small, locally run, free day-care nurseries or industrial crèches should be created so that mothers can return to work when they need to; fathers must be persuaded to take their family role as seriously as their work role; and employers must be persuaded to encourage this by allowing paternity leave and leave when children are ill; more research must be conducted into sociological, psychological and medical aspects of postnatal depression; all doctors, midwives, health visitors and social workers should be trained to understand and recognize the problem.

These are only a few suggestions; the reader will, I am sure, think of many others. All changes have to be fought for. But it will take time. Meanwhile women will continue to be depressed after birth, and the need for support and care will also continue.

It has, however, been heartening to find in the course of writing this book that the vast majority of people I have talked to have been concerned to find out about postnatal depression, have wanted to understand it and to know how they could help.

The most important way in which everyone can help is by openly discussing the problem and by admitting it exists, admitting, perhaps, that they have experienced it. By doing this we can relieve some of the shame attached to the experience and bring the whole subject of postnatal depression out of its underground darkness, up into the light of day to be examined. If this book can help to start such a discussion it will have achieved enough.

We must all stop blaming mothers for anything and everything that goes wrong in the lives of their children and recognize that women need to contribute their skills to the productive work of society and receive in return society's help and support with rearing *its* children.

References

1. Misconceptions

1 *The Baby Trap*, Ellen Peck (Heinrich Hanau, 1973).
2 *Character and the Conduct of Life*, William McDougall (Methuen, 1927).
3 *Any Woman Can!*, David Reuben M.D. (W. H. Allen, 1972).
4 Quoted from R. Stoller in *Sex, Gender and Society*, Ann Oakley (Temple Smith, 1972).
5 Joseph, 'Attitudes to work and marriage', quoted in *Housewife*, Ann Oakley (Allen Lane, 1974).
6 *Just Like a Girl*, Sue Sharpe (Penguin Books, 1976).
7 *The Captive Wife*, Hannah Gavron (Pelican Books, 1968).
8 *Children in Danger*, Jean Renvoize (Pelican Books, 1975).
9 *The Birth of a First Child*, Dana Breen (Tavistock, 1975).
10 *The Female Eunuch*, Germaine Greer (Paladin, 1971).
11 *Our Bodies, Ourselves*, Boston Women's Health Collective (Simon & Schuster, 1971).
12 *Patterns of Infant Care in an Urban Community*, John Newson and Elizabeth Newson (Pelican Books, 1965).
13 *The Birth of a First Child*, Dana Breen (Tavistock, 1975).
14 *Child Care and the Growth of Love*, John Bowlby (Pelican Books, 1953).
15 Quoted from *Our Bodies, Ourselves*, op. cit.
16 *A Woman on the Verge of Divorce*, Angela Reed (Nelson, 1970).
17 *The Baby Trap*, op. cit.

3. On the Road

1 Weissman, M. M., and Klerman, G. L., *Archives of General Psychiatry* 34, 854, 1977.
2 de Alarcon, J. G., Sainsbury, P., and Costain, W. R., 'Incidence of referred illness in Chichester and Salisbury', *Psychological Medicine* 5, 32-54, 1975.

3 Kendell, R. E., Wainwright, S., Hailey, A., and Shannon, B., 'The influence of childbirth on psychiatric morbidity', *Psychological Medicine* 6, 297-302, 1976.

4 Pitt, B., 'Atypical depression following childbirth', *British Journal of Psychiatry* 114, 1325-35, 1968.

5 Bardon, D., 'Puerperal depression', *Midwife and Health Visitor*, January 1972.

6 *Social Origins of Depression, A Study of Psychiatric Disorder in Women*, George W. Brown and Tirril Harris (Tavistock, 1978).

7 *Damned Whores and God's Police*, Anne Summers (Pelican Books, 1975).

8 *Immaculate Deception*, Suzanne Arms (Bantam Books, 1977).

9 *Idem.*

10 Quoted from *Giving Birth*, Sheila Kitzinger (Sphere Books, 1973).

11 Dr Duncan Dolton, Mersey Regional Health Authority specialist in community medicine, the *Guardian*, 10 December 1974.

12 *The Birth of a First Child*, op. cit.

13 Quoted in the *Sun*, 17 February 1975.

14 *Pregnancy, Birth and the Newborn Baby*, Margaret Mead (Delacorte Press/Seymour Lawrence, 1971).

4. First Steps in Alienation

1 Quoted in *Patterns of Infant Care in an Urban Community*, op. cit.

2 *Psychiatric Disorders in Obstetrics*, A. A. Baker M.D., D.P.M. (Blackwell Scientific Publications, 1967).

3 Quoted in the *Sun*, 17 February 1975.

4 Sabbagh, Sue, 'One in a hundred', *NCT Newsletter* 25, Autumn 1974.

5 *Communicating with the Patient*, P. Ley and M. S. Spelman (Staples Press, 1967).

6 *Human Aggression*, Anthony Storr (Pelican Books, 1970).

7 *Giving Birth*, op. cit.

8 *You and Your Baby*, Part I (BMA Family Doctor publication, 1977).

9 *Pregnancy*, Gordon Bourne (Pan Books, 1975).
10 Quoted from *Human Relations and Hospital Care*, Ann Cartwright (Institute of Community Studies, Routledge & Kegan Paul, 1964).
11 *Pregnancy*, op. cit.
12 *Human Relations and Hospital Care*, op. cit.
13 Moore, M. O., 'Antenatal care and the choice of place of birth', from *The Place of Birth*, eds. Sheila Kitzinger and John Davis (Oxford Medical Publications, 1978).
14 *Birth Without Violence*, Frederick Leboyer (Fontana Paperbacks, 1977).

5. Science and Technology

1 *Mary-Mary*, Joan G. Robinson (Fontana Lions, 1972).
2 Breen, Dana, 'The mother and the hospital', in *Tearing the Veil: Essays on Femininity*, ed. Susan Lipshitz (Routledge & Kegan Paul, 1978).
3 *Idem.*
4 Published in *AIMS Newsletter*, January 1978.
5 Cartwright, Ann, 'Mothers' experiences of induction', *British Medical Journal*, 745-9, 27 September 1977.
6 'Some mothers' thoughts of episiotomy', *AIMS Newsletter*, October 1977.
7 *Idem.*
8 *AIMS Newsletter*, October 1977.
9 *Truby King The Man*, Mary King (George Allen & Unwin, 1948).
10 'Fetal monitoring', *AIMS Newsletter*, 1977.
11 Quoted from Dawson, B. E., 'Orificial surgery, its philosophy, application and technique', in *The Anxiety Makers*, Alex Comfort (Nelson, 1967).
12 'Fetal monitoring', op. cit.
13 *Idem.*
14 Quoted in *The Psychology of Childbirth*, Aidan Macfarlane (Fontana Paperbacks, 1977).
15 Fielding, Waldo L., and Benjamin, Lois, 'The medical case against natural childbirth', *McCall's*, June 1962.
16 *Immaculate Deception*, op. cit.

17 *Brave New World*, Aldous Huxley (Penguin Modern Classics, 1955).
18 A midwife, quoted in the *Sun*, 17 February 1975.

6. *Birth and After Birth*

1 Kennell, J. H., Trause, M. A., and Klaus, M. H., 'Evidence for a sensitive period in the human mother', *Parent-Infant Interaction*, Ciba Foundation Symposium 33 (Elsevier Excerpta Medica, North Holland Associated Scientific Publishers).
2 *Human Relations and Hospital Care*, op. cit.
3 *The Psychology of Childbirth*, op. cit.
4 *Birth Without Violence*, op. cit.
5 Yalom, I. D., Lunde, D. T., Moos, R. H., and Hamburg, D. A., 'Postpartum blues' syndrome', *Archives of General Psychiatry* 18, 1, 16-27, 1968.
6 A personal experience quoted from *AIMS Newsletter*, September 1975.

7. *'I Remember, I Remember . . .'*

1 *AIMS Newsletter*, January 1978.
2 *Midwife and Health Visitor*, September 1974.
3 *AIMS Newsletter*, June 1976.
4 *Truby King The Man*, Mary King (George Allen & Unwin, 1948).
5 *Report of an Investigation into Maternal Mortality* (HMSO, 1937).
6 *AIMS Newsletter*, April 1978.
7 The *Guardian*, 12 May 1978.
8 Quoted by Margaret Whyte, organizer of the Society to Support Home confinements, *Spare Rib* 68, March 1978.
9 Gordon, J. E., Gideon, H., and Wyon, J. B., 'Midwifery practices in rural Punjab, India', *American Journal of Obstetrics and Gynaecology* 93, 1965; quoted in *Wisewoman and Medical Man*, op. cit.

10 Tew, Marjorie, 'Where to be born', *New Society*, 20 January 1977.

11 Cone, Brenda A., 'Puerperal depression', *Psychosomatic Medicine in Obstetrics and Gynaecology*, 3rd International Congress, London, 1971 (S. Karger, Basel, 1972), 355-7.

12 Tod, E. D. M., 'Puerperal depression – a prospective epidemiological discussion', the *Lancet* ii, 1264, 1964.

13 Ryle, A., 'The psychological disturbances associated with 345 pregnancies in 137 women', *Journal of Mental Science* 107, 279, 1961.

14 Pitt, B., 'Atypical depression following childbirth,' op. cit.

15 Dalton, K., 'Prospective study into puerperal depression', *British Journal of Psychiatry* 118, 689-92, 1971.

16* Hopkins, P., and Clyne, M. B., in *Modern Perspectives in Psycho-obstetrics*, ed. J. G. Howells (Edinburgh, 1972), 342.

17* *Psychiatric Disorders in Obstetrics*, A. A. Baker (Blackwell Scientific Publications, 1967).

18* Tylden, E., *Sunday Times*, 20 October 1974.

19 'The setting of childbirth and its effect on mother-neonate interactions', *Midwives Chronicle*, October 1974.

20 *Patterns of Infant Care in an Urban Community*, op. cit.

21 *AIMS Newsletter*, January 1977.

22 *Mothers and Midwives*, Claire Rayner (George Allen & Unwin, 1962).

23 *Limits to Medicine*, Ivan Illich (Open Forum, Marion Boyars Ltd., 1976).

* References given in 'Puerperal Sickness', a paper read by Dr D. Bardon at a National Course for General Practitioners on Psychosomatic Medicine – Life Events and Disease, Central Middlesex Hospital, 6 June 1974.

8. Father's Day

1 *Unmarried Fathers*, Dulan Barber (Hutchinson, 1975).
2 Quoted in *Women's Report* 6:4, June/July 1978, from *The Times*, 4 May 1978.
3 *You and Your Baby* (BMA Family Doctor publication, 1973).
4 Forbes, Ruth, 'The father's role', *Psychosomatic Medicine in Obstetrics and Gynaecology*, op. cit., 281-3.
5 Pawson, M., and Morris, N., 'The role of the father in pregnancy and labour,' *ibid.*
6 Lind, J., unpublished work, 1974, quoted by Kennell in *Parent-Infant Interaction*, op. cit.
7 *Mothering*, Rudolph Schaffer (Fontana Paperbacks, 1977).
8 Reported in *Spare Rib* 65, December 1977.
9 Miller, D. R., 'The world of women', *Psychosomatic Medicine in Obstetrics and Gynaecology*, op. cit.
10 *Sunday Times*, 14 May 1978.
11 'Changing childcare', *Spare Rib* 67, February 1978.

10. Cabbage Days

1 *Babyhood*, Penelope Leach (Pelican Books, 1975).
2 *Housewife*, op. cit.
3 *My Naughty Little Sister*, Dorothy Edwards (Young Puffin, 1974).
4 *The Captive Wife*, op. cit.
5 Richman, N., 'The effects of housing on pre-school children and their mothers', *Developmental Medicine and Child Neurology* 16, 53-8, 1974.
6 O'Reilly, Maria, 'Netherley united', *Spare Rib* 56, March 1977.
7 *Social Origins of Depression*, George W. Brown and Tirril Harris (Tavistock, 1978).
8 *The Captive Wife*, op. cit.
9 *Idem.*
10 Moss, Peter, and Plewis, Ian, 'Mental distress in mothers

of pre-school children in Inner London', *Psychological Medicine* 7, 641-52, 1977.

11 Ginsberg, S., 'Women, work and conflict', in *Mothers in Employment*, eds. N. Fonda and P. Moss (Brunel University, Uxbridge, 1976), 75-88.

12 'Mental distress in mothers of pre-school children in Inner London,' op. cit.

13 *Mothers: Their Power and Influence*, Ann Dally (Weidenfeld and Nicolson, 1976).

14 *Idem.*

15 *Feeding and Care of Baby*, Sir F. Truby King (Oxford University Press, 1945).

16 *Idem.*

17 *Mothers: Their Power and Influence*, op. cit.

18 'Mental distress in mothers of pre-school children in Inner London', op. cit.

19 Pitt, B., 'Atypical depression following childbirth', op. cit.

20 *Maternity: Letters from Working Women*, ed. Margaret Llewellyn Davies (first published 1915; Virago Books, 1978).

11. *'A Woman's Place is in the Wrong'*

1 Written by Sir F. Truby King in 1905, quoted from *Truby King The Man*, Mary King (George Allen & Unwin, 1948).

2 *Of Woman Born*, Adrienne Rich (Virago, 1977).

3 Quoted from the *Daily Mail*, 16 July 1977, in *Women's Report* 5 : 5, July/August 1977.

4 Quoted from the *Liverpool Echo* in *Spare Rib* 71, June 1978.

5 A comment made by Susan Brownmiller in *Against Our Will* (Secker & Warburg, 1975).

6 Quoted from *Pulse*, 8 April 1978.

7 'Mental distress in mothers of pre-school children', op. cit.

8 Quoted from a treatise by William Acton in *The Anxiety Makers*, Alex Comfort (Nelson, 1967).

9 Lomas, Peter, 'The significance of post-partum breakdown', in *The Predicament of the Family* (Hogarth Press, 1972). This particular quotation comes from an essay which is not otherwise insensitive to the wide range of factors involved in postnatal depression.

10 Lilith was the first wife of Adam who, according to the myth, refused to lie beneath Adam, claiming equality. When he tried to compel her obedience by force she rose into the air and left him, proceeding then to give birth to demons and populate the world with evil. From *Patriarchal Attitudes*, Eva Figes (Panther, 1970).

11 *Sunday Times*, 2 October 1977.

12 *The Hite Report*, Shere Hite (Talmy Franklin, 1977).

13 Silló-Seidl, G., 'The role of women in treatment of impotency', *Psychosomatic Medicine in Obstetrics and Gynaecology*, ed. Norman Morris (S. Karger, Basel, 1972).

14 *Alone of All Her Sex*, Marina Warner (Quartet Books, 1978).

15 *Domestic Medicine, or a Treatise on the Prevention and Cure of Diseases*, W. Buchan (Mitnel and Sowerby, Edinburgh, 1792), quoted in *Hard Labour*, Jean and John Lennane (Gollancz, 1977).

16 Based on statistics gathered by Dr Linda Fidell, Associate Professor of Psychology, California State University; 'Sex differences in health care', American Association for the Advancement of Science, 140th Annual Meeting, San Francisco, from *Off our Backs*, April/May 1975.

17 *Obstetrics and Gynaecology*, J. R. Willson M.D., C. T. Beecham M.D., and E. R. Carrington M.D. (Mosby & Co., 4th edition, 1971), quoted from *Off our Backs*, April/May 1975.

18 Zigmond, David, 'G.P. as therapist', *Mind Out* 26, Jan./Feb. 1978.

19 *The Birth of a First Child*, op. cit.

20 *Human Aggression*, op. cit.

21 *Depression*, Jack Dominian (Fontana Paperbacks, 1976).

22 *The Children on the Hill*, Michael Deakin (Quartet Books, 1975).

12. Private and Confidential

1 Bardon, D., Glaser, Y., Prothero, D., and Weston, D. H., 'Mother and baby unit: psychiatric survey of 115 cases', *British Medical Journal* 2, 755-8, 1968.
2 'Atypical depression following childbirth', op. cit.
3 Frommer, Eva A., and O'Shea, Gillian, 'Antenatal identification of women liable to have problems in managing their infants', *British Journal of Psychiatry* 123, 149-56, 1973.
4 *The Birth of a First Child*, op. cit.
5 *AIMS Newsletter*, January 1976.
6 One woman I talked to said her father used to tell her this.

13. The Black Rose

1 *The Archetypes and the Collective Unconscious*, C. G. Jung, translated by R. F. C. Hull (Routledge & Kegan Paul, 1969).
2 *Breast is Best*, Penny and Andrew Stanway (Pan, 1978).
3 Pitt, B., 'Atypical depression following childbirth', op. cit.
4 'Prospective study into puerperal depression', op. cit.
5 Tetlow, C., 'Psychoses of childbearing', *Journal of Mental Science* 101, 629-39.
6 *Human Aggression*, op. cit.
7 *Psychiatric Disorders in Obstetrics*, A. A. Baker M.D., D.P.M. (Blackwell Scientific Publications, 1967).
8 Pitt, B., 'Atypical depression following childbirth', op. cit.
9 *Human Aggression*, op. cit.
10 *The Vital Years and Your Child*, Audrey Bilski (Pan Books, 1973).
11 *Baby and Child Care*, Dr Benjamin Spock (New English Library, 1969).
12 Quoted in *Depression*, op. cit.

13 Protheroe, C., 'Puerperal psychoses: a long term study 1927-1961', *British Journal of Psychiatry* 115, 9-30, 1969.

14 'Medicine takers, prescribers and hoarders', *Social Studies in Medical Care*, Karen Dunnell and Ann Cartwright (Routledge & Kegan Paul, 1972).

15 Frommer, Eva A., and O'Shea, Gillian, 'Antenatal identification of women liable to have problems in managing their infants', op. cit.

16 *Of Woman Born*, op. cit.

17 Bardon, D., 'Puerperal psychosis', *Nursing Times*, May 1972.

18 Bardon, D., 'Puerperal depression', op. cit.

19 Bardon, D., 'Puerperal psychosis', op. cit.

14. Talk and Tablets

1 *Need Your Doctor Be So Useless?*, Andrew Malleson (George Allen & Unwin, 1973).

2 *Brave New World*, op. cit.

3 Foreword to 1946 edition of *Brave New World*, op. cit.

4 *The Female Eunuch*, op. cit.

5 Susie Orbach, quoted in '''omen's Talk' by Joy Melville, *Mind Out*, July/August 1978.

15. All Those Damned Hormones

1 *The Wise Wound, Menstruation and Everywoman*, Penelope Shuttle and Peter Redgrove (Gollancz, 1978).

2 *The Premenstrual Syndrome and Progesterone Therapy*, Katharina Dalton (Heinemann Medical Books, 1977).

3 *Postpartum Psychiatric Problems*, J. A. Hamilton (Mosby & Co., 1962).

4 'Birth of an Idea', Dr Colin Brewer, *The General Practitioner*, 28 July 1977.

5 'Prospective study into puerperal depression', K. Dalton, *British Journal of Psychiatry* 118, 689-92, 1971.

16. *In Conclusion*

1 A claim made by J. A. Hamilton for 'Traite de la folie des femmes enceintes, des nouvelles accouchées et des nourrices', by L. V. Marce (Paris, J. B. Bailliere et Fils, 1858) in his own book, *Postpartum Psychiatric Problems* (Mosby & Co., 1962).

Useful Addresses

The National Childbirth Trust
9 Queensborough Terrace
London W2 3TB

The Trust has branches throughout the country with antenatal teachers who run classes in prepared childbirth. They also organize postnatal support groups which help new mothers on a mother-to-mother basis.

Association for Improvements in Maternity Services (AIMS)
Secretary: Christine Beels
19 Broomfield Crescent
Leeds 6

AIMS is a birth pressure-group which seeks to ensure that the consumer's voice is heard and freedom of choice is retained. They are especially concerned about the modern tendency to streamline birth into standardized patterns. They are always more than pleased to hear from women about their experiences of the maternity services.

The Society to Support Home Confinements
Margaret Whyte
19 Tynedale Terrace
Newcastle-upon-Tyne 12

This group is working to reinstate the district midwife and retain the right for women to give birth at home. They will provide support for women who want to have their babies at home and provide information to counter arguments used by doctors.

National Council for One-Parent Families
255 Kentish Town Road
London NW5

Provides help and support for single mothers and their children as well as acting as a pressure-group to improve conditions for one-parent families.

Depressives Associated
Secretary: Janet Stevenson
19 Merley Way
Wimborne Minster
Dorset BH21 1QN

This is a self-help group run by people who have been depressed for people who are depressed. There are groups in different parts of the country and people who feel too depressed to attend group meetings are encouraged to write letters about their situation.

Women's Therapy Centre
6 Manor Gardens
London N7 6LA

This is a feminist therapy centre which is run on a voluntary basis by qualified psychotherapists. Group courses are included as well as individual therapy.

Meet-a-Mum Association (MAMA)
c/o Mary Whitlock
26a Cumnor Hill
Oxford OX2 9HA

A newly formed self-help group for mothers with babies.

Two useful pamphlets written by Margaret Dennis are available from the National Childbirth Trust:

The First Weeks of Motherhood
Guidelines for Counselling

Index

Sheila Kitzinger

WOMEN AS MOTHERS

How does a woman's behaviour change when she becomes a mother? Are there clear definitions of the 'right' and 'wrong' ways for mothers to behave? What kind of status do mothers now have in Britain and America?

In this wide-ranging study of motherhood, Sheila Kitzinger shows that maternal behaviour, far from being inborn and unchanging, is a direct response to the society the mother lives in. In closely-knit tribal societies, mothers will tend to keep their children with them all the time. In Western society, which places great value on independence and autonomy, every 'mother's aid' (pram, playpen, baby bouncer) is designed further to separate mother and child. Conception, pregnancy and childbirth itself are surrounded by quite different kinds of ritual and expectation, and Sheila Kitzinger examines the rituals of, for example, an American maternity ward and a birth in the African bush.

At a time when mothers in the West feel their role as an increasingly challenged and difficult one, and when women are re-examining their lives and status, Sheila Kitzinger's examination of one of the most important areas of a woman's life is illuminating and invaluable.

Edward Shorter

THE MAKING OF
THE MODERN FAMILY

How has marriage changed over the past three centuries? Is the nuclear family disintegrating, and why? Has women's new freedom affected the traditional sexual balance? And what is the role of children in the family, past and present?

In this remarkable history of the family in Western society, Edward Shorter draws on a wide range of research into such areas as courtship, illegitimacy, child care, sexual practices, family planning, and the sharing of household responsibilities. He describes not only changes in structure, but changes in how people, rich and poor, thought and felt about themselves. He shows how the Victorian 'sexualization' of marriage contributed to the development of the enclosed nuclear family, and suggests that in the future the couple, rather than the family, may be the key unit.

'a compulsively readable book' J. H. Plumb

'the material . . . is irresistible' Jonathan Raban

'vivid, admirably digested, immensely lively and full of ideas'
New Statesman

'A most important contribution to historical understanding'
The Times Literary Supplement

Katharina Dalton

ONCE A MONTH

Once a month, with demoralising regularity, over fifty per cent of women feel tired, confused, irritable and incapacitated due to the effects of premenstrual tension. Many others are indirectly affected – husbands, children, colleagues, workmates and friends.

Premenstrual syndrome is responsible for the timing of half of all criminal offences in women, for half of all suicides, accidents in the home and on the roads, hospital admissions, incidents of baby battering and alcoholic bouts. These are the calculable effects – how much greater are the less obvious changes in a woman's daily life, in her behaviour, appearance and health?

The problems might seem insurmountable – but are they? This book is a popular and easily understood account of menstrual difficulties by a doctor with many years of professional and research experience in their causes and treatment. Katharina Dalton shows that in most cases women can treat themselves, and that in severer cases progesterone treatment can be highly effective. It is a book which many readers – male as well as female – will find informative, sympathetic, helpful and above all practical in relieving the suffering caused by premenstrual syndrome.